IT'S N✱T ABOUT THE D🍴ET

Feel Strong and Alive
RIGHT NOW

DESIREE GREEN

HUGO HOUSE PUBLISHERS, LTD.

ISBN: 978-1-948261-22-7

Library of Congress Control Number: 2019916594

Cover Design & Interior Layout: Ronda Taylor, www.HeartWorkPublishing.com

Hugo House Publishers, Ltd
Denver, CO • Austin, TX
www.HugoHousePublishers.com

Printed in the United States of America

*This book is dedicated to two women that have shaped my life
into the loving, caring, praying, and nurturing woman
I am learning to become each day:
My mother Doris Goode and Aunt Georgine Smith.*

Contents

PART ONE—WHAT'S WRONG WITH ME?

CHAPTER ONE
Eye Candy 1

CHAPTER TWO
The Turning Point I Didn't Pay Attention To 5

PART TWO—THE MASTER GLAND OF THE METABOLISM

CHAPTER THREE
Why the Thyroid Gland is Important 13

CHAPTER FOUR
What Happens When Your Thyroid Doesn't Work. 21

PART THREE—FOOD IS MEDICINE

CHAPTER FIVE
My Mother and Food 37

CHAPTER SIX
The Food Plate Learning to Eat Healthily 43

CHAPTER SEVEN
Mindful Eating 53

CHAPTER EIGHT
Good Health Routines 57

PART FOUR—SPIRITUAL GROWTH

CHAPTER NINE
   Finding Strength in a Spiritual Path 71

CHAPTER TEN
   Letting Faith Guide Me .77

CHAPTER ELEVEN
   Get Moving! 81

CHAPTER TWELVE
   Getting a Divorce 87

CHAPTER THIRTEEN
   A Door Opens to A New Life 91

About the Author 95

"Self-Care is never a selfish act—it is simply good stewardship of the only gift I have, the gift I was put on the earth to offer to others."

—PARKER PALMER

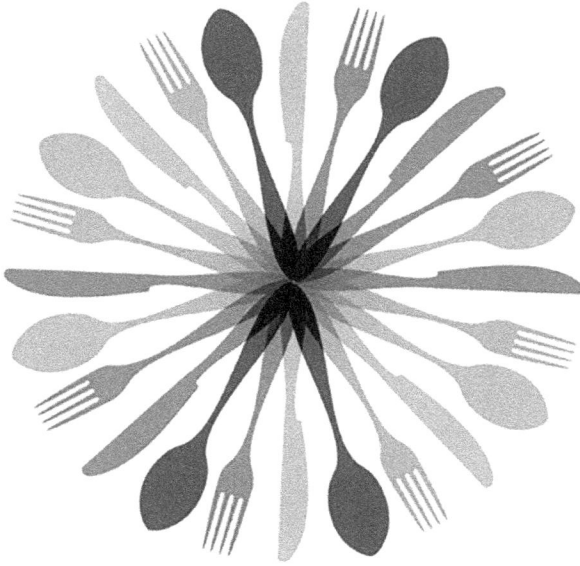

PART ONE

What's Wrong With Me?

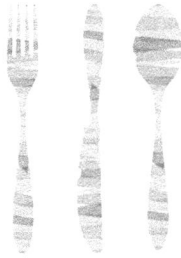

CHAPTER ONE

Eye Candy

EYE CANDY. YOU SEE A GUY (OR A GAL), WHO IS DROP-DEAD GORGEOUS. You make eye contact. They walk over. You have a drink. This person is a bit self-centered, but you ignore that little voice that says "don't do it," and you decide to have lunch. Lunch leads to dinner, which leads to …

What happens when it all goes wrong? You feel horrible. You wish you would have listened to that little voice and said, "you're something to look at, but this isn't going to work."

Have you ever looked at a brownie with intense desire, bathed in chocolate sauce and capped with a mountain of whipped cream (the real kind, the stuff you have to make yourself)? That's eye candy too.

That same little voice says, "don't do it," but you eat it anyway because it looks *sooooo* good. You take a bite thinking, "oh just one won't hurt me." You can't stop at one. And as you eat, your heart races, your blood pressure rises. That first bite tastes amazing. It probably even feels good—like the first time Mr. Eye-candy paid attention to you. But it doesn't take long for things to start going wrong.

This is your body saying "hello, not good." But because you don't know what to listen to, you keep eating.

That rise in blood pressure leads to a headache…then maybe light-headedness…then you crash because you're beyond fatigued, but you can't sleep.

Then you wonder, once again, why you can't lose weight, or why you have anxiety or feel depressed, or why you can't focus.

You feel like crap. So you eat more things that are bad for you because they make you "feel" good, but then when the initial effect wears off (and sometimes that can be within minutes), you feel even worse.

Is this you?

Common Problems Dieting Won't Fix

How many of you can't lose weight no matter what you do?

You think, "If only I could lose fifteen pounds (or twenty, or fifty), I would feel so much better about myself."

Maybe you have the opposite problem. You can't gain weight, and you're tired of looking like a bean pole. People who need to lose weight don't get it. They think, "but you're thin, how can you be unhealthy?" They don't notice how tired and depleted you look all the time.

The complaints we have about our bodies are common—almost frighteningly so.

It gets worse. Sometimes you feel like everything is moving so fast, but no matter how much you think, "I need to keep up," you can't. But maddeningly, you also can't relax. Everything feels like it's on hyper-drive, like you're over-amped. Your body is exhausted, but your mind is racing—constantly. It's like the storm you can't get out of. You feel foggy, and there's a lot of confusion.

Sometimes it feels like you're in a total disconnect. But no amount of rest, no amount of ice cream, or caffeine, or alcohol, or pizza—or any of the other "comfort" foods or stimulating drinks we have come to rely on—get you anywhere.

What about body temperature? You're always too cold, no matter what the temperature. Either that or you get too warm or even hot, and nothing seems to work to cool you down.

If you get a panic attack, you feel like everything is closing in on you. You can't catch your breath. Your head feels like it's about ready to explode, and you feel unsteady on your feet.

The doctors can't quite figure out what's wrong with you. You go multiple times to multiple doctors, and because they can't figure it out, they recommend medical drugs—or worse, psychotropic, mind-altering drugs. You take them, but they don't really work. The medical drugs actually make you even more physically sick. The mind-altering drugs make you feel like a zombie, like you can't feel. The worst part is you don't feel like *you*.

You go back to your doctor, and he or she does what doctors do: if medication doesn't alleviate the symptoms (never mind fixing the problem), then they recommend you get surgery or something else extreme.

Then it's a life-time of medication to compensate for the body part they removed. Never mind that you will never again feel exactly right. And here's the worst part: you still have the same symptoms.

That is how I lived my life for twenty-two years. I was living with far too much stress. I wasn't eating the right foods, and I certainly wasn't paying attention to the bigger spiritual part of myself.

This is not the life I want for you.

Through a major overhaul of how I approached life—both in the way I handle problems as well as the way I eat—I was able to overcome the major health issue I had developed.

I want you to understand not only what happened to me, but what you can do *now* so that you don't have to experience anything extreme. My desire for you is simple. I want you to make better health decisions for you.

What follows is practical advice that I wish I had known even ten years ago, because if I had, I would have made different decisions about my health. I wouldn't be living in a constant search for ways to make up the damage I allowed the doctors to do to me.

What I am going to impart to you isn't always the easiest path. We have been trained to think that all we need to do is "take a pill" for whatever ails us—physically or emotionally. But a pill very rarely handles the underlying issues.

The fact is we got ourselves into the shape we're in in large part by the food and drink we've put in our mouths. So the way to fix it lies in the same realm. You can't eat a bunch of processed food, or fried food, or even a lot of wheat and sugar (and for many of us, dairy), and wash it down with too much alcohol and not have some health implications. What you eat and drink has a huge impact on your health and how you feel.

However, to say that this is a diet book would be a misnomer. It goes beyond that, because I realized, as I was working through my own issues, that food is energy, but there's also the energy that we surround ourselves with. This is the energy—positive or negative—that comes from the people we associate as well as the way we feel about ourselves, our bodies, our minds, *and* our spirits. It's the two energies together—the physical and the spiritual—that we need to be mindful of and use to help ourselves heal ourselves and find a happier, balanced life.

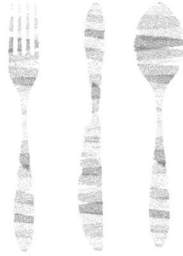

CHAPTER TWO

The Turning Point I Didn't Pay Attention To

I N THE EARLY 2000'S MY LIFE SEEMED ON TRACK. I WAS A THIRTY-YEAR OLD mother to my nine-year old and one-year old adoring sons and thriving in my career as a supervisor for the government. But I had issues—the same ones I described in the previous chapter. I couldn't gain weight. I was tired all the time. I had anxiety—a lot.

In late 2003, I was diagnosed with thyroid disease. The doctor told me I had a goiter. I had no idea what that meant at the time or that things I had experienced all my life might relate to this condition. A "goiter" is by definition an enlargement of the thyroid gland. (The word, interestingly enough, comes from the Latin word for "gullet" or throat. It has nothing to do with the gland itself.) Most people have heard of the thyroid gland, but very few know why it's important. My doctor didn't. He also didn't say anything about what caused that condition. Turns out, that was the most important thing to know.

My thyroid had swollen to a point that it was "unsightly."

That was actually the main reason my doctor gave me why I should consent to having my thyroid removed. It is "unsightly," but that's the least of your worries.

I was like most people. I really had no idea what it was. I definitely had no clue what it did or how vital a healthy thyroid is to overall good health.

I do know that I always felt like my life was moving fast, and I could not slow it down. I struggled with focusing on tasks and completing assignments.

My family considered me the "flaky" child. School was a struggle because I could not focus on assignments. I did not do well in school. My last year of high school, the teacher told my mother I had to go to summer school. My mother was not happy and told me to figure it out because summer school was not an option in her house. The next semester, I took as many classes as possible to the point I had no lunch. I was able to graduate on time. It didn't get better the older I got. I had to train myself to focus in college by sitting still for hours reading and finding fun ways to study.

Mornings were a struggle for me as well. I was *always* tired. I would wake up with headaches and body aches. I dreaded waking up because I felt like a truck ran me over twice, and I would stay in bed for at least an hour trying to get myself together for work.

Every winter I had a cold or the flu without fail. I started to get used to this inevitability and prepared myself with a cabinet full of cold and flu medications. None of them ever stopped me from having the illness—they just made the symptoms bearable when I got sick.

I secretly struggled with depression and never feeling smart or good enough. Thank God for my religion; prayer helped me through those thoughts.

When I got diagnosed with thyroid disease, my doctors told me that I needed to monitor the growth of my thyroid, but I didn't need thyroid medication.

None of the doctors told me how to actually take care of my thyroid. In fact, they didn't even explain what the thyroid is (I do that in the next chapter.)

There was no information anywhere on how food, exercise, or lifestyle might help regulate my thyroid. Nor did they ask me any questions about some of the conditions I suffered, like being unable to gain weight, depression, confusion, and spaciness. These I later learned are very much related to thyroid function.

I didn't take the diagnosis seriously and didn't educate myself on thyroid disease—the first of many mistakes. My focus was on being the best mother to my sons and having the best career. I could take medicine for the condition—problem solved. Or so my thinking went.

For seven years, I ignored the swelling in my throat. Finally, in 2010 I decided to have my thyroid removed. I have to admit, it *was* unsightly, having a big bulge in my throat. It also made it tough to swallow, even breathe sometime.

But then tragedy struck twice in my life–my healthy seventeen-year old son contracted a life-threatening illness, and my dear mother got cancer, all within 2010 to 2012. So much for taking care of me.

While coping with these tragedies, I finally had my thyroid gland removed My mother flatly refused to go to the doctor unless I did something about my condition. The result was worse than the problem. I suffered disastrous health consequences that the doctors didn't prepare me for. They certainly didn't give me any information on how to cope.

What kept me going was my belief in God. God led me down the path I eventually took of natural healing and learning to love myself enough to take care of my body, mind, and spirit.

Because God gave me a chance to make it right, I have written this book to share my story with others who feel like they're going crazy. It is important to listen to your heart. If something doesn't feel right, then it probably isn't.

It Really Isn't All About "The Diet"

We go on all sorts of diets: the traditional low calorie/low fat diet; low carb/high protein; ridiculously low carb and high fat; eating a grapefruit before each meal; eating what our ancestors ate; eating food according to your blood type. Each diet is touted as the "miracle diet," and it works for some. For others, it doesn't. My friend is a Type A blood type. She's supposedly able to eat grain—preferably whole grain according to that protocol—legumes and other starchy foods. She laughs at the thought. If she ate everything on the "approved" list, she would be as "big as a house," as she says.

Losing weight is not about just going on a diet and "watching what you eat." Gaining weight is definitely not about eating anything you want—which usually includes sugary, processed foods that are full of empty calories that your body can't use.

Getting to and maintaining a healthy weight really isn't "all about the diet," when you're thinking "diet" in the usual sense—restricting calories, eating low-fat foods, eating "diet" processed food that you can get at the grocery stores.

I talk to a lot of people—men and women—about their diet. There are many of them who are unhappy with how they feel—tired all the time—and really frustrated that they either can't lose weight or gain it. But I find they are unwilling to give up the very things that are making them that way, the sugar, dairy, wheat, and processed food. It tastes good. It's their comfort food.

I get it. I wish there was a magic pill that would allow us to eat that chocolate brownie with the home-made whipped cream and chocolate sauce on top.

But your ability to live well—with energy and verve—has never come from a pill. First, it very much is all about using food as medicine, knowing what foods will help your system handle the health issues it is facing (like my thyroid issue) and avoiding foods that make your body weak and bloated with inflammation. This requires change—change in your dietary habits, how you approach food, and the mindset with which you tackle all of life.

If you ask any of my doctors, they will tell you that my thyroid problem is purely physical. However, I learned—and continue to be reminded—that true good health is a matter of living a decent life. That has helped me handle my thyroid issues far more than the synthetic thyroid hormones the doctors have prescribed for me.

My Mission–Finding Balance for a Healthy Life

Living well means finding balance in your life. Finding balance, however, is not about waking up every morning and feeling "balanced." Too many of us wake up feeling like everything is out of balance. So we strive to balance everything in your life. If you look at balance this way, you don't set expectations that you can reach.

First, "finding balance" is not static. You don't reach some middle ground and say, "That's it. I found balance." Finding balance is knowing you have to make decisions that will come in line with your will to live a healthy life right now. There is no end point as long as you are living, but the great thing about finding balance is you get better each day at achieving your goals!

Finding balance is a revolving door because there will be things and people that will shift your foundation and make you readjust. We call that transition. I am constantly telling my clients, "Transition is never easy, but sometimes it is necessary."

Now, there are good transitions like the birth of a child, graduation, marriage, etc., and there are negative transitions. For me, transition came in many of these forms, but the negative transition for me was death, divorce, and sickness. They both matured me and helped me grow as an individual.

Growth can be positive or negative. It can make you withdraw from life and forget all the good qualities you have to give to life to thrive and live a balanced life. This is one of the main reasons people eat in an unhealthy way; they don't feel worthy.

This is why I have become a health coach. Being a health coach is not all about nutrition. I leave that work for the nutritionists. Health coaches help the client realize and support what they need to balance their lifestyle and wellness. We help you understand your bio-individuality, meaning, what works for you as an individual.

The majority of my struggles came from my inability to express myself and keeping things inside. It caused my digestive system to shut down. The way I was living—keeping things shut inside, doing what I'm supposed to but not feeling positive about it—would never have allowed me to find a way to heal my digestive system. I didn't know how to express myself and let go. Once I learned to express myself and release my pain, I started to make choices that I was comfortable with in my life and eating towards those goals.

My life experience coupled with my health-coach training has set me on a path of success! There is not a person I have encountered who asked for my help that I didn't assist in changing their life. I love what I do because it is who I am.

It is a blessing to be able to share my experiences with my clients and watch them reevaluate their lifestyle choices and make adjustments that help them find balance.

I want to be able to help you in your journey towards feeling strong and alive (not weak, overwrought, anxious, and crappy)—right now!

Are you ready?

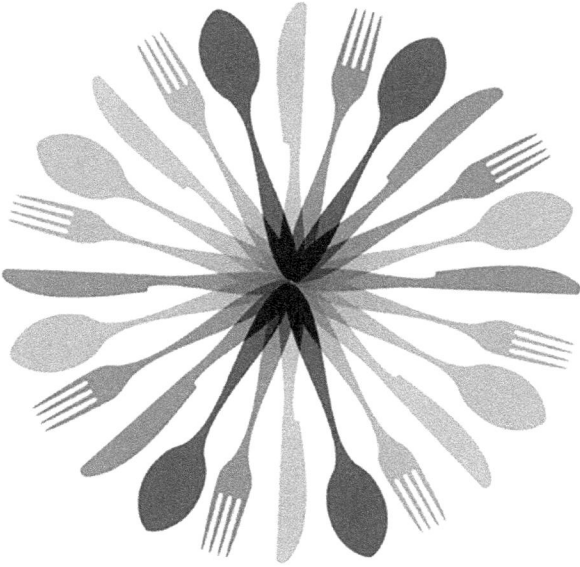

PART TWO

The Master Gland of the Metabolism

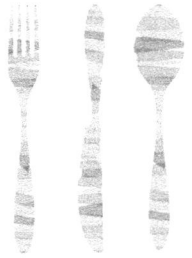

CHAPTER THREE

Why the Thyroid Gland is Important

WARNING: THIS IS VITALLY IMPORTANT. IF YOU'RE SUFFERING FROM all the symptoms I listed in the previous chapter, you get medical attention concerning your thyroid immediately:

❖ losing or gaining weight
❖ not being able to regulate body temperature
❖ feeling anxiety or depression
❖ not being able to focus
❖ feeling "over-amped" or like you can't slow down
❖ being exhausted or fatigued all the time but you can't sleep and never feel rested

If that medical attention includes a health coach and alternative medicine treatments, then more power to you. It means you want to take charge of your health in positive, proactive ways!

What is the Thyroid Gland

In Part One, I told you how I was diagnosed with an enlarged thyroid gland (the "goiter") and ultimately had it removed. According to the doctors, that should have handled my problems. But it didn't. It made them worse. Why? Because when they removed my thyroid, they actually removed a vitally important part of my body.

Because no one told me what this thing called a "thyroid" is or why it's so important, that's what I'm going to do right now!

The entirety of this chapter is to help you understand what the thyroid is and what it does, so you understand better why I keep talking "thyroid," when I'm talking about health issues.

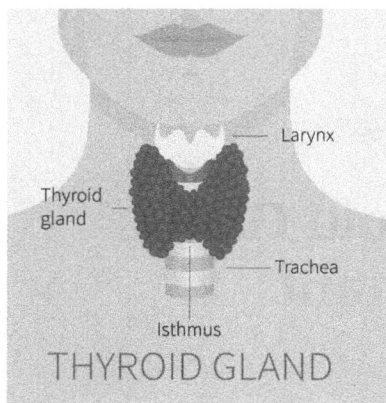

The thyroid is about a two-inch butterfly shaped gland at the base of your throat. A "gland" is simply a sack in your body that builds up different kinds of fluids and discharges that fluid either directly into the blood stream (like in the case of the thyroid) or onto an internal surface (like the pancreas secreting digestive juices) or external surface (like sweat glands).

When a gland isn't doing its job properly, it is either stopped up and not secreting enough of the fluid it's supposed to, or it's secreting too much. Think "over active sweat glands." Your body is secreting too much sweat out of those glands.

Glands are all over your body, doing various jobs to keep our bodies up and running smoothly, and they secrete all kinds of fluids, like digestive fluids.

The fluid that our glands secrete most into the blood stream contain chemicals called hormones. Most people know "hormones" as the sex hormones that can make you go nuts over Mr. Eye Candy and lose all sense of good reason. I will dive into hormones later in this chapter, but for now, just know that the thyroid is vitally important for the regulation of hormones in your body.

Thyroid Issues

Thyroid issues are far more prominent than people think. One study shows that one out of seven people, or close to 15 percent of the population, suffers from thyroid disease and they don't know it. That means a *lot* of people have *major problems* with their thyroid like mine. Far *more* people have thyroid issues that cause problems that aren't technically classified as disease. Their thyroid is either secreting too much or not enough of the hormone it's supposed to. And that causes a whole world of hurt—either way.

As I noted in the previous section, a goiter is simply an enlargement of your thyroid. You should never have to wait for a goiter to develop. It means that your thyroid has not been working properly for a very long time. If the goiter is in the early stages, unless you have been diagnosed with thyroid cancer, you should research other options before surgically removing the goiter.

It is far more effective to start treating the condition early, at the first signs of trouble.

Thyroid issues are more prominent than most people realize because the thyroid affects so many functions in your body. But because I waited so long to treat my thyroid disease, it felt like I finally had no choice but to remove the gland.

After the surgery, my health declined rapidly. I suffered constantly from headaches, body aches, colds, toothaches, panic attacks, and *erythema nodosum* on my legs. *Erythema nodosum* is a type of skin inflammation that is located in a part of the fatty layer of skin. *Erythema nodosum* results in reddish, painful, tender lumps most commonly located in the front of the legs below the knees. There were days I couldn't get out of bed because of the pain.

They never said that this is what happens when you lose your thyroid gland and that these are issues that happen when your body is unable to regulate hormones. They just kept prescribing pain meds and antibiotics, and not one of my doctors at that time said anything about what I could do proactively to stabilize my hormones; simple things like changing my eating habits and exercising more.

In spite of all these problems, the doctors, including my endocrinologist couldn't find anything "wrong with me." So the doctors did what they often do—prescribe more medication. They told me to take more pain meds, which only made me feel dull and unmotivated. And because I was constantly sick, even though I don't think I had a bacterial infection, the doctors just kept prescribing antibiotics and steroids, which didn't work. In fact, these medicines probably did more harm than good because my gut flora (the "good bacteria" needed for digestion) was constantly being killed off.

Finally, my doctor referred me to an arthritis doctor. He diagnosed me with osteoarthritis. This is where the cartilage degenerates and breaks down, which causes joint pain and stiffness. I was going from bad to worse, and to compound it all, my mother passed away. I was thirty-nine years old. I felt like I was ninety, and I was quickly descending from grief into apathy. I was ready to give up and allow my illness to get the best of me and become a slave to medications—medications that would have deadened me spiritually and ultimately killed me spiritually.

But I didn't. I decided to get educated instead.

I asked the doctor how I could stop the progression of the arthritis. He indicated that I needed to exercise more—finally, a doctor who was dispensing some common sense.

But the problem is, while exercise can help arthritis, what he didn't tell me was that certain foods could cause inflammation and inflammation causes arthritis—and if I really wanted to handle the condition, I had to pay attention to what food I was putting in my body. I didn't learn this until later on in my health journey.

But at least it was a start.

Why is the Thyroid So Important?

People often talk about the thyroid in relation to weight—most of the time if they can't lose any. I was familiar with that idea, but since I've been a bean-pole most of my life, I didn't think that was an issue for me. Boy was I wrong.

The thyroid is related to weight issues, but how does it function, and why is it called the "master gland of the metabolism"?

There are so many misconceptions about the thyroid gland. Too many. So I've decided to take you through my learning process on why the thyroid is so important. What follows is how I took the deep dive into figuring out what the thyroid is and what it does. And more to the point, once you know what you're dealing with, then you can decide (like me) how your thyroid is affecting your body.

Here goes…

My Search

The thyroid gland, according to the Everyday Health Website:

> "helps control your metabolism and other important bodily functions (everything from helping your body to regulate temperature to the desire for intimacy)."

Right off the bat, I get that there's two parts to what the thyroid does:

1. It controls how energy is used in cells (that's metabolism), and

2. It controls other important bodily functions. But I had to pause. I've always been told that my metabolism was really fast, and those who have put on too much weight suffer from a slow metabolism.

But I had to ask myself, what is "metabolism"? It's a word we've all heard hundreds of times, but what does it really mean?

Well, MedicineNet defines metabolism as

> "the whole range of biochemical processes that occur within a living organism. Metabolism consists of anabolism (the buildup of substances) and catabolism (the breakdown of substances).
>
> The term metabolism is commonly used to refer specifically to the breakdown of food and its transformation into energy."

This is a lot of information for my mind to process. I have to break it down into plain language for me to understand the meaning.

This is what I discovered. We are a living organism that requires energy to live. MedicineNet indicates the energy we require is food because food transforms into energy.

So our thyroid has to do with how we convert and use energy in our body. While the research shows the physical aspects of that, I had to wonder about the other forms of energy and their effect on the thyroid.

I believe that there are different kinds of energy. Food is where we get our physical energy; however, I believe energy also comes from quality of life (social, spiritual, relationship, etc.). It takes all types of energy: physical, emotional, spiritual, and even mental energy to create the biochemical processes we need as living organisms.

But no matter how our energy manifests itself, I was finally beginning to see why this little butterfly-shaped organ that is two inches long near the base of the neck is so important. It's managing the energy balance in your body!

This is good news for you, but I am sad for me. My doctor didn't educate me on any of this. I wish he had *before* he told me that I needed the "goiter" removed.

Everyday Health goes on to say the thyroid "releases hormones that help control your metabolism and other important processes in the body."

Okay, there's that word again: hormones. What does it really mean?

Hormones

MedicineNet states, "a *hormone* is a chemical substance produced in the body that controls and regulates the activity of certain cells or organs." The energy we take in is distributed by our hormone system.

Okay, so the thyroid gland, which regulates metabolism, does so through these substances called *hormones.*

It finally made sense why my health declined so rapidly. Because I no longer had a thyroid, I no longer had a way to manage the energy in my body. My body was no longer able to distribute the energy my body was producing through digestion correctly. And because I no longer had a thyroid, *all* my hormone levels (not just those that were produced and regulated by the thyroid) were way off, something the doctors neglected to inform me would happen.

Endocrine System

But I had to step back even further. If all my hormone levels were off, then my thyroid must be connected to other parts of my body. That made me ask: what are the organs that are controlled by hormones? Well, they are all part of the endocrine system.

The **endocrine system** is the collection of glands located throughout the body. It is a system that consists of the majority of your organs "that produce, store, and release hormones into the bloodstream."

The endocrine system consists of the hypothalamus, pituitary gland, thyroid, parathyroid, adrenal glands, pineal body, reproductive glands, and pancreas. These glands produce over fifty different hormones that regulate almost all the functions in the body! These glands and the hormones they secrete regulate metabolism, growth and development, tissue function, sexual function, reproduction, sleep, and mood, among other things. (And you thought that hormones were only involved in sex.)

Here are just two examples of the hormones that you're probably familiar with. The pancreas regulates insulin—when that goes out of whack, the person has diabetes. The adrenal glands secrete adrenaline. If a person is constantly in a stressful situation, the adrenal glands secrete too much adrenaline and other hormones (primarily cortisol), and that causes havoc on the body.

What's most important to know is that these glands are all in a "system," which means that all these glands in the endocrine system are connected. They all work together as a whole.

Unfortunately, we're lead to believe these hormone factories work solo. They don't. When you remove an ovary or a thyroid, other parts of the system don't work as well because each part of this system can no longer communicate with each other. It is similar to losing a love one you can no longer call and talk to about your problems, and they used to help you with a solution.

My body was no longer producing essential hormones and because a major part of my endocrine system was removed, it now made sense why I was experiencing all those problems. A major part of that inter-connected system was *gone*.

> *I cannot stress this enough: it is not a pleasant way to live when you're missing a major part of your endocrine system. Your body is constantly trying to compensate, trying to make up the damage that cannot be undone. There are effective alternatives to surgery, and I urge you to do research, seek out an alternative-care health practitioner, and take the necessary actions to keep your organs and glands intact. The reward is simple: the potential for a longer, healthier, more active life.*

In Plain Language

I just threw a bunch of terms at you—hormones, metabolism, endocrine system. If you're like me, you need things to be broken down into plain, common-sense language.

This is how I put it all together:

The energy we take in, which could be food or quality of life, speaks to the chemicals in our body which are called hormones.

Based on the information the hormones receive, the hormones will then work to balance the body.

The balance comes in the form of our digestion, metabolism, growth, reproduction, and mood control. Yes, mood control!

I will talk about the food you eat all throughout the rest of this book, but how many of you have indulged in "stress eating," when you eat anything because you're really stressed out, upset, sad, or even depressed?

The energy we take in is transformed into the hormones in our body which then is regulated by the metabolism, and based on the energy (good or bad) it shows up in our health. All of this works closely with our nervous system—the system in our body that helps all the parts of our body communicate with one another.

But think about this: your mood is controlled by your quality of life, and that drives the food you eat. The source of your mood is how you react to the world. This comes back to energy!

What if you could go to the doctor, and he or she prescribed just walking away from all the negative energy that you are consuming? By doing this, you could be giving your body the space in which to change your metabolism and hormones? If you have had that experience, please give me that doctor's number!

It shocks me that western medicine is still compartmentalizing our health. For example, you have a headache, you take a pill. The pill (usually aspirin or ibuprofen or even the latest craze with Cannabidiol—CBD— oil) deadens the pain. It's doesn't treat the cause of the headache. Therefore, you're not getting healthier by taking pain medication.

To get healthy requires that you pay attention to how the body functions as a whole. Remember in the last section when I talked about balance? It starts with balancing your hormones—as many of those fifty as you can—by helping those endocrine organs secrete them properly and at the right time. That action helps balance metabolism—and while a lot of you girls think you would like a "fast" metabolism, that causes its own problems. What you're going for is a balanced metabolism.

And above all, you're going for a balance of energy in your life—handling the negative energy, bringing on the good positive energy, and moving forward with verve and vigor—with life!

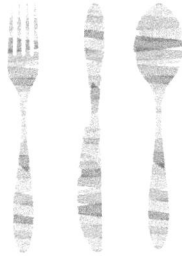

CHAPTER FOUR

What Happens When Your Thyroid Doesn't Work

THERE'S A PILL ON THE MARKET THAT IS BASICALLY SYNTHETIC THYROID hormones. It's touted as a sort of "cure all" for thyroid glands. It does help regulate your thyroid gland, and if you are like me with no thyroid, it is needed.

But I have issues with the "take-a-pill" approach. One, taking a "med" for something that ails you rarely if ever solves the problem—even if that is the favorite way a doctor solves a medical issue these days. As I said in the previous chapter, it usually only serves to either get rid of a symptom, which doesn't solve the underlying issue. Or it simply masks the problem. That's not a solution, either.

If you have a thyroid issue (or other glandular problems like diabetes), why take a pill that's synthetic and suffer unhealthy and unpleasant side effects when you can regulate your thyroid (or pancreas or other organ in the endocrine system) by understanding and treating the underlying cause?

Let's go back to the idea of balance. If a function in your body is not balanced with other functions in your body, then you get symptoms: cold hands and feet, swelling or bloating, constipation, headaches. You name something that doesn't feel right or "good" with your body, and you can usually trace it back to an imbalance of at least one function but probably a number of them.

Inflammation

Inflammation has been the big buzz word lately in both the traditional and alternative medicine fields. Inflammation is the body's way to heal itself by fighting injury and infection. It's an amazing immune-system response that must work well in our bodies. However, chronic inflammation (when the immune-system response continues over time and long past when it was useful) can trigger or even cause many unwanted conditions. For example, it may be an underlying cause of cancer.

Inflammation is when the white blood cells rush to an area, flooding that area in order to remove the problem. This response protects us from infection, bacteria, and viruses. Without this immune response, we would have no way of fighting disease.

But the problem happens when that immune response gets out of balance.

Inflammation is like a light switch; it can be easily turned on. There are many factors that can trigger this response: food you're sensitive or allergic to or stress that doesn't go away. Also, your lifestyle behaviors can cause the switch for inflammation to be turned on.

Causes of Inflammation

Food

There are many processed foods that can cause inflammation. For example, saturated fats, Trans fat, Omega 6 fatty acids, refined carbohydrates, MSG, and alcohol. We'll go into food in much more depth later. For now, just remember that food is what gives your body physical energy, but if you're not eating healthy food, or are eating food that your body reacts to, then it can cause inflammation.

Anxiety and Depression

One of the most common causes of inflammation is anxiety and depression. And yes, an out-of-balance thyroid can do the same (and if you're starting to make that connection, good for you!)

Anxiety can hit anyone, but it is most common in woman and young adults. If you worry about everything, you could be suffering from anxiety disorder. It is important to seek some sort of counseling (and don't discount the counseling offered by your Church), to help you manage your anxiety.

I had a therapist who helped me mange my fears and taught me techniques to stay calm under pressure. Anxiety is an inner-emotional conflict between yourself and the outside world. It can cause responses in your body that make you react to the food you're eating. This can send you down a dark road and cause you to lose control which will send your blood pressure into levels unknown.

When my son fell sick, I had an anxiety attack every day. It had gotten so bad my legs began to swell and break out in big blotches below my knee—the *erythema nodosum*, which I noted before. It was so painful. I couldn't walk and had to see a doctor. The doctor did what doctors do, gave me a "pill," in this case steroids, and sent me home. After careful research, I learned that *erythema nodosum* is caused by inflammation.

I had to learn to manage my anxiety and deal with life one step at a time. It's not easy, which is why I suggest you seek professional help (and don't discount the help your church can give you), but it is worth it!

Depression is not the same as anxiety. Please do not confuse the two because the outcome is different. Depression is a feeling of failure. Nothing pleases you. With depression, you feel tired all the time and have no energy to participate in anything. You can't sleep, your appetite is minimum to none, you feel helpless, and you have thoughts of death or suicide. Depression can cause you to avoid eating and taking care of yourself. When you are depressed, you deprive the body of the nourishment it needs to thrive.

I think we all deal with depression in some way or other—who hasn't at some time felt like they didn't want to get out of bed or deal with life? The difference is to what degree have they been depressed?

There are many effective non-medical ways to treat depression. A good diet and exercise can sometimes work miracles. I learned, in order to handle depression, I had to do some work on me. I needed to understand my purpose in life. You can do the same. Write your purpose down and keep it all around the house. It will remind you of your worth and the foundation of who you are in life and your purpose.

Next, build your self-esteem. I have an app on my iPhone for affirmations. Every day, I receive a different affirmation that helps build my self-esteem. I read that affirmation out loud throughout the day.

Lastly, honestly assess your health and how it relates to your emotional need. If you are dealing with a health issue, identify it and deal with it by seeking out help to understand how it is emotionally impacting your life. The physicians and other caregivers will treat your physical ailments without addressing your emotional need. Don't be afraid to ask your doctor for help to address your emotional needs as well. If your doctor is unable to help you in this way, then I highly recommend finding a doctor that is open to working with a wellness center. I am starting to see a growth in medical practices incorporating wellness centers, so hopefully it will be easier for you to find a good holistic doctor that can address you more fully as a person (not a symptom!).

8 Indicators of Inflammation

Chronic inflammation leads to rheumatoid arthritis, atherosclerosis, periodontal disease, and hay fever. It can cause heart disease and diabetes. Remember how I was diagnosed with osteoarthritis? It was because basically I had too much inflammation in my joint areas. My father suffered from rheumatoid arthritis his entire life. I know others who have been crippled by the problem.

Headaches are another indicator of inflammation—a huge one. They were the cause of one of my biggest struggles before getting healthy.

There are many names for headaches, but for me, it was a migraine, tension, and clusters.

My journey into better health has taught me the difference between these types of headaches. A tension headache has nothing to do with emotional tension even though we want to blame it on our kids and husband. A tension headache is painful contractions in the head, neck, shoulders, and face. It causes a tightening feeling around the head. Lack of sleep would trigger my tension headache. I make it a must to get enough sleep each night. However, whenever I have a tension headache, I immediately drink lots of water and do yoga. I stretch out and relax those areas to relive the pressure.

A migraine and cluster headaches are different beasts. My son and I used to suffer severely with migraine headaches. It would force us to a dark room for days. Painkillers did not help ease the pain. We had to wait it out. If I only knew that it was because of inflammation.

Migraines and cluster headaches are vascular headaches. "Vascular" refers to the vessels that carry the blood. Think about it; if it is vascular, the vessels must be constricted which is causing lack of blood to the brain. This sounds dangerous. A migraine is intense and stays around for days, and clusters come and go for hours. Either way, you are dealing with a vascular issue. This could be caused by some incident. For me, it was food.

Once I started the better health journey, I started to learn sodium was poison. The minute I had sodium, it would send me straight into a migraine, especially Monosodium glutamate (MSG). I am careful to read the labels on my food, and I find it safer to cook fresh. I will delve in–depth into food in Part 3. For right now, the point is simple: even major issues like migraines and cluster headaches can be handled with a change in your diet.

For now, think about what we've gone through: the endocrine system is responsible for making sure your body is physically in balance. It can be thrown off by both physical and mental energy that's bad—bad food, bad moods, bad/toxic people.

Inflammation is an indicator that something isn't right in your body. It means that your immune system is over-reacting, and that causes severe problems.

And yes, there is a very direct connection between inflammation, the organs in the endocrine system, and a body that's out of balance. For example, diabetes is caused by inflammation of the pancreas, the organ which produces the hormone insulin. This is because inflammation is the direct cause of a health problem that is becoming more known and understood: autoimmune disease.

Autoimmune Response and Disease

The immune system is protecting you from the dangers of infections and disease. What happens when your immune system turns on you and starts attacking the healthy cells in your body? Well, you have an autoimmune disease.

My family has a history of autoimmune disease—and I know that we're not alone. According to WomensHealth.gov, more than 23.5 million Americans are affected by autoimmune disease.

"Autoimmune" means that the immune system has turned on itself and starts to attack healthy cells. That's the "response" part of the equation. When that happens a lot, then you have "disease."

According to the same article in WomensHealth.gov, the immune system has the ability to tell the difference between what's supposed to be there and what's foreign. However, when there's a flaw, the immune system fails to differentiate, and the immune system attacks normal cells by mistake. At the same time, other special immune system cells called "regulatory T cells" fail to do their job of keeping the immune system in line. This causes the immune system to attack your body. WomensHealth.gov says that "the body parts that are affected depend on the type of autoimmune disease. There are more than eighty known types."

Eighty is an alarmingly large number of "known types" of autoimmune diseases. Diseases that have been typically very hard to treat, like psoriasis, lupus, and rheumatoid arthritis (as I mentioned above), are all autoimmune diseases.

Unfortunately, I know too much about this subject.

There is no real explanation for how autoimmune can occur. MedlinePlus online states "They do tend to run in families. Women—particularly African-American, Hispanic-American, and Native-American women—have a higher risk for some autoimmune diseases."

There are many factors that can trigger an autoimmune disease. There is a great chance, although it hasn't been proven, that the foods you eat that are processed (food that has been altered from its natural form), high in trans-fat, and loaded with sugar and salt, could have a significant impact on autoimmune disease.

Think about it, processed foods are chemically-altered foods, and you are putting them into your body. When chemicals are added to the food during the processing (and if you need any proof of that, read the list of ingredients on a bag of cheese puffs—pick any brand), those chemicals like the dyes and preservatives, are going straight into your body. We won't mention the herbicides and pesticides that are used on most of the food we eat.

Then we have the chemicals in your house, for example cleaning products, detergents, hygiene products, etc. Every day, we are exposing ourselves to chemicals, and they can cause your body to go out of balance and ultimately cause this autoimmune reaction.

Autoimmune disease has only within the last decade become a "household" idea. Fifteen years ago, you wouldn't have heard or read about a connection between the immune system attacking itself and diseases like diabetes or lupus. As such, it's not as well-researched as "say" heart disease. Scientists can't pinpoint the exact mechanism that causes it. That doesn't mean that it doesn't exist or that the effects are very real and hugely detrimental.

Thyroid Problems: an Autoimmune Response

What has this all got to do with the thyroid? I can tell you this: unless your thyroid gland has been removed or deformed at birth, thyroid issues are almost if not always autoimmune issues.

And there's the connection my doctors didn't tell me but one I so desperately needed to know.

The thyroid is the "master gland of the metabolism." When it isn't functioning properly, the metabolism isn't working properly. This is why a person gains weight or can't put on weight. It's also why a person gets cold hands and feet. The body isn't maintaining its internal temperature—it can't burn fuel or it burns too much fuel. The energy needed for warmth is not there, so the body gets cold.

There are two very well-known thyroid issues:

Hypo-thyroidism—this is when the thyroid is not producing enough thyroid hormones. The most common form of this is something called "Hashimoto's Disease" (after the surgeon in Japan who discovered it in 1912) and is a known auto-immune disorder."

Here is a list of symptoms of Hashimoto's:

❖ Fatigue and sluggishness

❖ Increased sensitivity to cold

❖ Constipation

❖ Pale, dry skin

❖ A puffy face

❖ Brittle nails

❖ Hair loss

❖ Enlargement of the tongue

❖ Enlargement of your thyroid gland (goiter)

❖ Unexplained weight gain

❖ Muscle aches, tenderness and stiffness

❖ Joint pain and stiffness

❖ Muscle weakness

❖ Excessive or prolonged menstrual bleeding (menorrhagia)

❖ Depression

❖ Memory lapses

Hyper-thyroidism—this is when the thyroid is producing *too much* of the thyroid hormones. This is what I suffered from, and as you will see, the goiter is one of the symptoms.

❖ Anxiety and irritability

❖ A fine tremor of your hands or fingers

❖ Heat sensitivity and an increase in perspiration or warm, moist skin

❖ Weight loss, despite normal eating habits

❖ Enlargement of your thyroid gland (goiter)

❖ Change in menstrual cycles

❖ Erectile dysfunction or reduced libido

❖ Frequent bowel movements

❖ Bulging eyes (Graves' ophthalmopathy)

❖ Fatigue

❖ Thick, red skin usually on the shins or tops of the feet (Graves' dermopathy)

❖ Rapid or irregular heartbeat (palpitations)

I can't imagine anyone saying "Wow, I want to have unexplained weight gain" or "Being depressed is fun!" or "You know, I think having thick, red skin on the tops of my feet is sexy."

So let's put this all together: your thyroid is the gland that basically regulates your physical energy. When it has too much inflammation in it, then it starts attacking itself—that's the autoimmune response. This causes all these extremely bad, unpleasant things to happen in your body.

Not good.

The Thyroid Hormones

The thyroid's main job is to produce two specific hormones, and these hormones help regulate all sorts of things: breathing, heart rate, muscle strength, cholesterol levels, and body temperature.

Your thyroid uses your energy to produce iodine. This is why iodine was added to salt—it was specifically to prevent goiters. (No kidding.)

Iodine is an essential trace element that your body can't produce on its own, but it is essential to thyroid health. It is the element that helps your thyroid creates two hormones: Thyroxine (T4) and Triiodothyronine (T3). They are so named because of the number of iodide molecules—T4 has four and T3 has three. Pretty simple.

Let's start with T4, thyroxine. T4 is the inactive form of the thyroid hormone. It is produced in far greater amounts than T3—around 90 percent more. Why? Because when the T4 reaches organs and body tissues, it converts into T3 (Triiodothyronine), which is the active form of the thyroid hormone. That's the form that tells your body how to use energy.

T4 is the stepping stone to get T3. If your body doesn't produce enough T4, then it can't make enough T3—and that's when you get hypothyroidism (Hashimoto's). If you are producing too much T3, then you get hyperthyroidism (Graves.).

The obvious fix here is to make sure you get a decent amount of iodine. A health practitioner I know recommends potassium iodide and iodine.

But there's actually more to it.

How the Endocrine System Connects

The thyroid also controls your body's sensitivity to other hormones.

Remember when I told you about the endocrine system? It's a tightly connected system of glands, and your thyroid isn't acting alone. Far from it.

It actually goes back to the pituitary, the gland that is the overall "master gland." It's the "master" because it controls the other main glands in your body—the adrenals, ovaries and testicles, and the thyroid (of course.)

The pituitary gland produces something called TSH, or Thyroid Stimulating Hormone. TSH is what stimulates production of both T4 and T3 in the thyroid gland.

Now, just to make things more interesting, right above the pituitary gland, which is a pea shaped gland just below the bridge of your nose, is the hypothalamus. This is a small but mighty organ that the Pituitary Foundation describes this way:

> "The hypothalamus serves as a communications center for the pituitary gland, by sending messages or signals to the pituitary in the form of hormones which travel via the bloodstream and nerves down the pituitary stalk. These signals, in turn, control the production and release of further hormones from the pituitary gland which signal other glands and organs in the body.
>
> The hypothalamus influences the functions of temperature regulation, food intake, thirst and water intake, sleep and wake patterns, emotional behavior and memory."

Wow! When I first read that, I needed to figure out what it said. So, again in simple language: the hypothalamus talks to the pituitary gland through the use of hormones. Those hormones send messages to other glands in the body to "do their thing," and produce their hormones.

This really helps me understand how connected this whole system is and why making sure the glands that produce and secrete all those hormones stay healthy. The hormones are the messengers—without them, our bodies don't know what to do or how to act properly.

Endocrineweb makes it even clearer:

> "the hypothalamus produces TSH Releasing Hormone (TRH) that signals the pituitary to tell the thyroid gland to produce more or less T3 and T4 by either increasing or decreasing the release of a hormone called thyroid stimulating hormone (TSH)."

When levels of T4 or T3 are low, the pituitary tells the thyroid to produce more hormones. When your levels are high, the pituitary tells the thyroid to produce fewer hormones.

If the pituitary is out of whack, then it's not telling the thyroid to produce more hormones or shut off its hormone production for a while.

I created this diagram to help me understand the logic behind the thyroid. It is not scientific or anything professional. It is my thoughts on paper, and I am sharing it with you in the hopes it will help you understand.

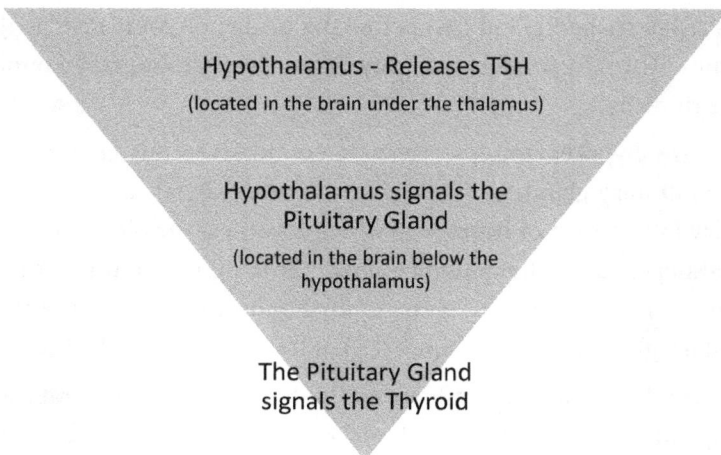

Hypothalamus - Releases TSH
(located in the brain under the thalamus)

Hypothalamus signals the Pituitary Gland
(located in the brain below the hypothalamus)

The Pituitary Gland signals the Thyroid

This whole system is set up to produce either more or less Thyroid stimulating hormone (TSH), which then signals the thyroid to produce more or less T4 which is then converted into T3.

So what does all this mean?

First, we need to pay attention to the entire endocrine system because it's all connected. Yes, this book is about keeping your thyroid healthy, but doing that also means keeping the pituitary and the hypothalamus functioning properly as well.

Second, if your body is experiencing inflammation, which triggers the autoimmune response, then the glands that produce the hormones that tell your body how what to do are either going to produce too much or too little of those hormones. That wreaks an unbelievable amount of havoc on your body because those hormones tell your metabolism what to do. Remember, metabolism is the breakdown of food into energy. If I put this all together in my mind, it means allowing bad energy into your body (food or lifestyle) will eventually cause your immune system to attack your thyroid. Wow!

We don't want that. So how do you know what hormones your body is producing and to what degree?

Fortunately, this is where the medical doctors come in handy. There are tests that can show how much or how little of the T4 hormone is in your body. But you do need to ask for them.

Thyroid Antibody Tests

The problem with doctor visits is that they don't routinely check your thyroid levels unless there are signs of an abnormal thyroid function. As for me, it was only tested when the presence of a goiter showed up. I believe if I had been tested early, I would have known my immune system was attacking my thyroid and I could have taken measures to reverse the attack.

There is a series of tests that you need to ask for if you suspect you have thyroid issues. It's all about testing for the thyroid antibodies.

Thyroid antibodies are a test performed to understand the autoimmune disease and to "distinguish it from other forms of thyroid dysfunction."

Thyroid antibodies are formed when "the immune system mistakenly targets components of the thyroid gland or thyroid proteins, leading to chronic inflammation of the thyroid, tissue damage, and disruption of thyroid function." You should recognize that as a description of autoimmune disease.

Which Test to Ask For

Lab Test Online provides the following test to establish a diagnosis.

❖ Thyroid peroxidase antibody (TPO)—the most common test for autoimmune thyroid disease; it can be detected in **Graves disease** or **Hashimoto thyroiditis**.

❖ Thyroglobulin antibody (TGAb)— this antibody targets thyroglobulin, the storage form of thyroid hormones.

❖ Thyroid stimulating hormone receptor antibodies (TSHRAb)—includes two types of autoantibodies that attach to proteins in the thyroid to which **TSH** normally binds (TSH receptors):

◆ Thyroid stimulating immunoglobulin (TSI) binds to receptors and promotes the production of thyroid hormones, leading to **hyperthyroidism**.

◆ Thyroid binding inhibitory immunoglobulin (TBII) blocks TSH from binding to receptors, blocking the production of thyroid hormones and resulting in **hypothyroidism**.

The next time you go to the doctor, make sure they perform *all* of the above blood tests. Having all of these tests performed initially will help you understand the cause of the attack on your thyroid. This can help you know which measures you need to start taking to reverse the immune system attack on your thyroid. TBII is a test you must ask for because doctors most likely will not perform this test.

The Lab Test Online provides a great chart of when thyroid test is performed. See opposite page:

THYROID ANTIBODY	ACRONYM	PRESENT IN	WHEN ORDERED	OTHER FACTS
Thyroid peroxidase antibody	TPOAb	Hashimoto thyroiditis; Graves disease	When a person has symptoms suggesting thyroid disease; when a health practitioner is considering starting a patient on a drug therapy that has associated risks of developing hypothyroidism when TPO antibodies are present, such as lithium, amiodarone, interferon alpha, or interleukin-2	Has been associated with reproductive difficulties, such as miscarriage, pre-eclampsia, premature delivery, and in-vitro fertilization failure
Thyroglobulin antibody	TgAb	Thyroid cancer; Hashimoto thyroiditis	Whenever a thyroglobulin test is performed to see if the antibody is present and likely to interfere with the test results (e.g., at regular intervals after thyroid cancer treatment)	
Thyroid stimulating hormone receptor antibody, Thyroid Stimulating Immunoglobulin	TRAb, TSHR Ab, TSI	Graves disease	When a person has symptoms of hyperthyroidism	

Notice, it is not a routine procedure to have your thyroid checked. I am not sure why because understanding early if your immune system is attacking your thyroid is important in reversing the attack and treating the condition.

I went for health checks regularly for years prior to having my thyroid removed. I never discussed thyroid issues with my doctor—even though I was experiencing hyperthyroid symptoms regularly—and my blood work was always good. Well, it wasn't until I was presented with a goiter that my doctor started looking at my thyroid, and even then, my thyroid levels were normal.

One last bit of advice. I read a lot of articles on thyroid disease and health, and one article I thought important to share was Dr. K. News (www.drknews. com/unraveling-thyroid-antibodies/)

> "When I have a patient who is struggling with symptoms of both hyperthyroidism and hypothyroidism, a strong indication of Hashimoto's, and the antibody test comes back negative, I run the second panel. Because the autoimmune response waxes and wanes, the patient may test negative one week and positive the next. Sometimes I may even ask the patient to enjoy extra sugar and gluten in their diet before the second test, as sugar will drive up inflammation and gluten will provoke the autoimmune response, both of which better the chances of producing a positive result on an antibody lab panel."

In other words, if you are having symptoms (fatigue, weight gain/loss, constipation, cold intolerance, muscle aches and pains, depression—the same list of symptoms I began Part Two with) and your levels are normal, don't stop. Stay on your doctor to continue running more tests. You are not crazy. What you are going through is real!

You want your body working optimally. That's when you feel alive, energized, ready to take on the world, and create the life you want. If your body doesn't respond that way, then instead of taking a pill for whatever symptom you're dealing with, work to balance the function that's stopping you. This requires some attention and determination, especially because the best "medicine" you can give your body is the food you eat. So the next stop on this train to good health is all about what you are feeding your body.

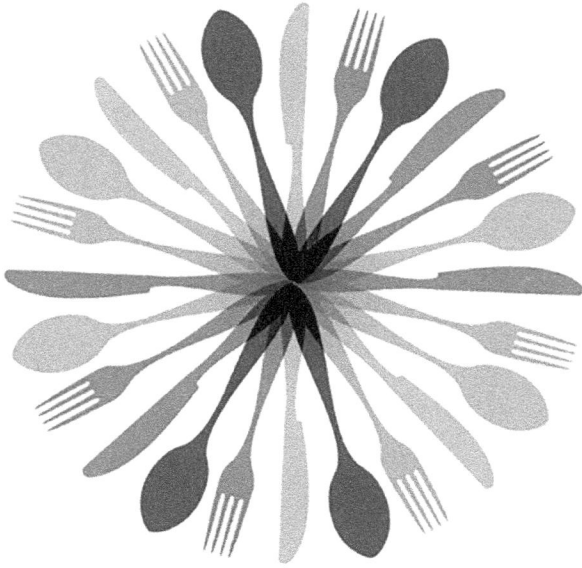

PART THREE

Food is Medicine

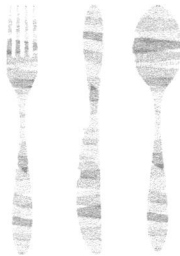

CHAPTER FIVE

My Mother and Food

L ONG BEFORE I ENDED UP HAVING MY THYROID REMOVED, I KNEW I NEEDED to find another path. The pills, the steroids—they didn't work, and I didn't want to take them. I was determined to learn all I could about food and health. I had no idea what path to take. So, I decided to hire a health coach. Best decision of my life. She opened my mind to a whole new world.

After a few months of working with my health coach, I felt better and could clearly see the difference in eating healthy food. But then my work schedule got crazy and I was traveling much more. My work schedule had me flying between Los Angeles and New York almost twice a month. My sons also took up a lot of attention—attention I was very willing and happy to give. The older one was on medication that I had to teach him how to use. My youngest son was signed up for baseball, basketball and football: every time the seasons changed, the sports changed. I was too busy with life. I had an idea of what I should be doing, but truth be told, I was not really taking care of me. Then tragedy struck. My mother was diagnosed with esophageal cancer. My life was thrown in turmoil.

I'm starting this section on food with my mother because she was a woman full of life and the kitchen was a part of the fabric of her heart. More than anything my mother loved cooking and especially for her family. She was the house you went to for Sunday dinner—any dinner to be honest.

She expressed her love and caring for us by giving us a full course meal every time we walked in the door. Many times my friends would come to my house for a home-cooked meal because they couldn't get one in their home. Happily my mother cooked for us all as a way of providing a safe haven for my friends.

Her cooking was amazing! She could take any kind of food and make it into a delicious meal. Her southern cooking could be smelled out the door, down the stairs, and across the street. All you had to do was follow the trail.

The esophagus is the tube that starts at the end of your throat and continues to your stomach. It is the pipe through which everything you eat and drink travels. Because hers was cancerous, my mother was unable to eat and enjoy the very thing that gave her life. She had basically stopped eating and had lost a tremendous amount of weight.

Before she would go see a doctor, she made me get my thyroid removed. I had the surgery, and there went the hormone-producing machine that my body so badly needed to help regulate so many systems in my body, including my mood. But I did it so my mom would go to her doctor, get the treatment she needed, and would stop worrying about my health.

My mom's doctor suggested giving her a feeding tube before starting chemotherapy and radiation. After surgery for the feeding tube, she had a stroke.

This devastated my family. My mother was the matriarch. My mother passed away a few months after my surgery, in 2012.

Her death was extremely stressful for me, and I'm still recovering. I had lost my mother, I was also having to take care of my son who had just received a heart transplant (more on that in a bit), and I was struggling with the aftermath of losing my thyroid.

If it wasn't for my health coach and what she taught me, my hormone levels would have been so wacky I would have been hospitalized. If I were hospitalized, who was going to take care of my sons? Realizing this pushed me further into learning how food and the body relate.

I loved my health coach because she never made me wrong about what I ate. She gently coaxed me, showing me how to prepare food and what were the best foods to keep me healthy. Her gentle touch lives on with every person I help because I know how valuable that support was for me.

Unfortunately with my work schedule, all my responsibilities and my mother's illness and death, I had to eventually part ways with my health coach. And when I did, I thought I didn't have the time or patience to follow the plan my health coach provided for me. It didn't take me long to start suffering the consequences of that choice. That's the nice way of saying that I realized that I made a really dumb decision. My body quickly fell apart.

I wasn't doing well, so I decided that I better do something drastic—follow my health coach's advice, no matter what, and do my own research. It was at that point that I decided that I wanted to help others as my health coach had helped me, and from that point, I quickly conceded that I needed to go from being my own worst enemy to my very best client.

What follows is what I learned and the way that I now help others.

Food as Medicine

Remember when I said there are other, highly effective, alternative ways to treat not just physical ailments but mental issues like depression. One of the most effective I have found to be food!

As the subtitle states, food is medicine. What you put into your mouth that eventually makes it into your system as energy can hurt you very much or it can help you immensely.

The typical American diet is chock full of food that is known to cause inflammation. Remember, inflammation can lead to autoimmune disorders and disease, hypo- and hyper-thyroidism among them.

My mother cooked your typical southern style. Cornbread loaded with butter, bacon grease the staple fat, and everything—and I mean *everything* had sugar in it. I didn't know what food tasted like without sugar, to be honest.

Sugar, dairy, red meat, processed food, and gluten-laden grains were my staples. Those are what most Americans eat, and yes, those are the problem foods that cause inflammation.

That's why the chocolate-sauce drenched brownie with whipped cream—the one I talked about in the introduction—the one that looks sooo good and tastes even better does such a number on you when you eat it.

It causes all those important glands in the endocrine system to become inflamed. The inflammation then causes the gland to either not produce enough of the hormone it is supposed to or too much. And I don't have to go over again the long list of body problems that causes.

So here's the question. If food got you into that trouble, doesn't it make sense that food will get you out of it?

The simple answer to that is yes. My health-coach taught me that.

Food really is some of the best medicine we can take. Dr. James S. Gordon, a psychologist who touts alternative therapy for mental health, tells the story of his mentor, Shyam Singha, who was a London-based Indian osteopath, naturopath, herbalist, acupuncturist, homeopath, and meditation master. At one point, Dr. Gordon was told he needed back surgery. Instead, he asked his mentor for advice. Dr. Singha told him to eat "three pineapples a day for a week," and nothing else. It worked. Dr. Gordon didn't need back surgery.

It is now well-known in alternative health circles that the five main foods that cause the most problems are gluten, dairy, sugar, meat that is raised on GMO foods (like corn and soy), and processed food. Those are also the hardest foods to eliminate from our diet because they taste good. They make up so much of our "comfort food."

I lost my mother to cancer because she ate "comfort food," her whole life. I don't want that to happen to anyone else.

Part Three is all about the food we eat. Yes, I am suggesting that you change the way you eat—maybe even radically. And I'm not talking about what you usually think about "diet." Remember, food is energy, and you want to be putting the best energy-producing foods in your body. Food that causes inflammation doesn't do that.

An anti-inflammation/auto-immune diet is not always an easy one to follow. However, the alternative to me is *far* worse.

I may say this until I'm "blue in the face," but having to deal with wacked-out hormones all the time because I don't have a thyroid is not something I would wish on my worst enemy. Do you want to lose an important organ like your thyroid? Or end up with diabetes because your pancreas doesn't work? Or get cancer because you have chronic inflammation and your body can't kill the cancer cells.

If you have answered no to any of those questions, then it's time to make the decision to change what you eat, even how you eat, so you can have more energy and feel alive. Who doesn't want that?

The Anti-Inflammatory Diet

I'm going to dive right in.

I suggest you start with the elimination diet by Dr. Axe. If you are not sure what is causing the inflammation, the elimination diet is great because it is not a long-term plan. You remove foods from your diet and slowly reintroduce the foods one at a time to determine which food is causing the inflammation. However, I also recommend removing or minimizing processed foods even after you do the elimination diet. Just Google "Dr Axe Elimination Diet," or go to this link: https://draxe.com/elimination-diet/

Then, start following an anti-inflammatory diet, also called an auto-immune diet.

Some of the best out there include *The Autoimmune Solution* by Amy Myers, MD (my editor and publisher, who also has had to deal with inflammation issues, swears by this one), and *The Plant Paradox* by Steven R. Gundry, MD.

I personally like *The Anti-Inflammatory Diet Cookbook* by Madeline Given, NC. It provides great recipes and a list of healthy choices and foods to avoid. The recipes come with some educational information on how it will help the body.

Foods to Avoid

Madeline Given gives you foods to avoid (the list of Foods That Worsen Inflammation), and it is a very standard, accepted list:

- ❖ Fats and oils
  - ◆ Margarine
  - ◆ Oils: canola, corn, peanut, rapeseed, soybean, vegetable
  - ◆ Trans fats (often called hydrogenated or partially hydrogenated oils on the ingredients label)
- ❖ Nuts and Seeds
  - ◆ Peanuts
- ❖ Grains
  - ◆ Corn, genetically modified (i.e., not organic per the USDA's National Organic Standards, or verified non-GMO by a third-party organization like the Non-GMO Project)
  - ◆ Refined wheat flours
  - ◆ Wheat and other gluten-containing grains; barley, bulgur, farro
  - ◆ Wheat pasta

- ❖ Unfermented Soy Products
  - ◆ Soy: beans, milk, protein, sauce
  - ◆ Vegetable protein, textured
- ❖ Citrus Fruits (in excess)
  - ◆ All
- ❖ Nightshade Vegetables (if sensitive to them)
  - ◆ Eggplant
  - ◆ Peppers
  - ◆ Potatoes, white
  - ◆ Tomatoes
- ❖ Feedlot Meat and Animal Products
  - ◆ Dairy products, processed
  - ◆ Eggs, factory-farmed
- ❖ Sweeteners
  - ◆ Agave nectar
  - ◆ Sugar: brown or white, refined
  - ◆ Syrup: corn, high fructose corn syrup

The rest of Part 3 is all about how to incorporate that list into something that works for you. However, don't beat yourself up if you have some ice-cream at your daughter's birthday party. Dr. Gordon, the guy who ate pineapple for a week to keep from having back surgery, has some very good advice. He reminds us not to become a "food fanatic." This list of foods that cause inflammation offer you a guideline. If you do happen to have a "cheat day" and eat something you're not supposed to (like some amazing French bread loaded with butter), it's okay. He says, "Just notice the effect of a questionable choice, learn, and return to your program."

Food is energy, and energy is life. Learn what works for you, and enjoy the benefits of making good food choices.

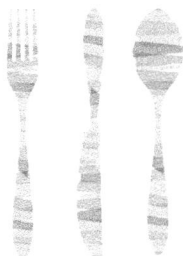

CHAPTER SIX

The Food Plate
Learning to Eat Healthily

W HEN I WAS TAKING HEALTH COURSES TO BECOME A CERTIFIED HEALTH
coach, I learned about the "integrative food plate." There are many
versions of it, but the basic idea is that you use your plate to portion your
food in percentages (kind of like the pizza with which you used to learn about
fractions like half, quarter, thirds, and eighths when you were a kid.)

It's a good idea overall, and you can search the internet to find various
examples of it. But learning to eat healthy comes down to one very important
rule: eat what you know is good for you.

No matter what you eat, however, it should include a large portion of vegetables. Veggies that are cooked or raw—however your body likes them—should
be *the* staple in your diet. The only way *not* to eat veggies is if they're canned.
The canning process takes all the nutrition out of them.

After veggies, then it really is what works for you. Most integrative food
plates that I've seen are ¼ fruits, ¼ veggies, ¼ protein, and ¼ nuts, seeds, and
grains. But what if your body can't digest grain, soy, nuts, and seeds? What if
you react to fruit? You can tell what works by how you feel—just make sure to

incorporate a *lot* of veggies (my editor, who can't digest seeds, nuts, and grain, says her food plate is ¾ veggies and ¼ protein. She eats fruit maybe once a week, and she steers clear of the grains, nuts, and seeds. She eats around nine cups of veggies a day and the benefits are clear: she sleeps better and her whole digestive system is working better than it ever has.)

If you're not eating the right things, your mind and body are disconnected. There's no conversation going on in your body between your body's organs and between you and your body. You want the conversation to be happening, and you want to be able to listen to it. You know when it's happening because your body is responding to what you put it in.

Journaling what you eat everyday eventually becomes your own personal diet. That's what I did, and now I have a specific diet that I know works for me.

The human body is a machine and what you put in that machine determines how well it will perform. If you fuel it with junk food, processed food, and GMO food, you will have a machine that will always break down and not perform well.

Unfortunately, we cannot buy a new body. It may work better to take care of the body God gave us by fueling the body with fresh veggies, fresh fruits, and cooking healthy dishes.

Here are some additional food tips that I help people with all the time:

Try New, Healthy Foods

My health coach taught me the importance of cooking all my food fresh rather than eating fast food. She introduced me to many different, healthier cooking alternatives, and broadened my perspective on food.

I had never been a cook. That was my mother's love. I ate. By learning to cook, I began to greatly enjoy cooking. I was learning something new about myself, and it brought me closer to my mother.

At first, my cooking was similar to my mother's style of cooking. I would cook collard greens with pork, baked mac and cheese with several different kinds of cheese, and more. But my health coach taught me it's healthier to bake and when I cooked to use healthy oils, for example, olive oil or coconut oil and not to deep fry. She never criticized me for my style of cooking. She only provided suggestions.

Though I had learned much from my health coach, I still didn't fully know exactly what constituted good and bad food. When I read *Integrative Nutrition*, I learned much more about dietary guidelines, genetically modified organisms (GMOs), the danger of processed foods, the need to eat seasonal foods, identifying cravings, and more.

Most importantly, I came to understand how food can be your medicine or your poison. As I have noted above, I wanted it to be my medicine as much as possible.

Eat What Your Great Grandmother Ate

Most of what we eat in the Standard American Diet is processed food. This food is bad for us. Food that is processed contains synthetic flavoring, preservatives, chemicals, and dozens of other food additives. Hot dogs, lunch meat, all "junk food" like chips and cookies, even cooked vegetables in a can, are all processed.

The food industry doesn't much care because all these chemicals and additives make the food look and taste good, so we buy more. Profit is their goal, and they care less that such "false" food lacks the nutrition our body needs to function and that makes us sick.

Did you know that up until around 120 years ago, it was rare for people to die from heart disease, strokes, cancer, and autoimmune diseases like M.S., or diabetes, Alzheimer's, and Parkinson's? People began to die from these lifestyle diseases when we switched from food from the earth to unnatural and processed foods.

For years, I suffered from digestive issues that caused acid reflux and nausea. I was miserable. I know now that much of this came from all the processed food that I was eating. Processed food confuses our body which doesn't know how to process this unnatural food. Our digestion system was designed for foods that the earth supplies for us. When we eat false and unnatural food, we feel sick, put on weight, become fatigued, suffer digestive disturbances, get depressed and spacey, and have trouble sleeping all because our brain isn't being fed,.

For thousands of years, human beings ate nothing but what the earth supplied—organically grown fruits, vegetables, seeds, nuts, and meat. If you want to live a long, healthy life, you need to revamp your grocery list. Buy fresh, raw *not* processed food. That's some of the very best medicine you can buy.

Eat from the Earth

Remember, food from the earth is not processed. To be truly healthy, try to load up on the following food:

❖ Fresh fruit

- Non-starchy vegetables (carrots, celery, cucumber, spinach)
- Starchy root vegetables in moderations (squash, sweet potatoes)
- Cruciferous vegetables, broccoli, cauliflower, kale, peas
- Nightshade plants in very small amounts (green pepper, eggplant, tomato, white potato)
- Not-gluten grains like buckwheat, millet, quinoa, rice (jasmine and basmati are the best in my opinion) and non-GMO soy
- Nuts
- Legumes
- Non-pasteurized dairy products
- Free range meat or organic

I want to talk a bit about eating organic eggs. When I first started eating healthy, eggs were a part of my diet. But I didn't know the difference between cage-free and pasteurized eggs. I bought eggs!

Now that I was learning so much more, I was now careful to buy only organic pastured eggs (not "free range" or even "cage-free." I learned that cage free eggs could still mean the hens are inside but not in cages. It is important the package reads "pastured."). With organic pastured eggs, hens are cage free and can roam, spread their wings and lay their eggs **in nests**.

In contrast, most commercially produced eggs come from hens **confined in** cages and never go outside. "Free Range" means that they have access to the outdoors for a limited time each day. You don't know if the chicken ever took advantage of that. Being caged in this way affects their behavior and the hormones that course through their systems. It also affects what they eat.

Rather than nibble on the grass outside, caged hens are given mostly corn and gluten grains to eat. Such grains might also contain lots of additives that are not listed on the packaging. These additives include pesticides to keep the feed "clean," as well as additives to increase immunity in flocks, to increase the nutrition or shell-strength of eggs, and even alter the color of the yolk. This is more unnatural stuff we put into our bodies with potential ill results!

In general, make it a rule to stay away from refined grains (white bread, enriched white pasta), processed foods (cake, candy, cookies, chips), white potatoes, sweetened soft drinks, and sugar (especially refined sugar.) The only exception to this is white rice—it has been shown to be less inflammatory than brown rice.

These are bad foods not only because they are likely to be genetically modified but because of how they upset your blood sugar level and make you jumpy. They break down quickly in your bloodstream and flood it with glucose or simple sugars. This causes a quick release of the hormone insulin, causing your blood sugar to spike and making you feel edgy.

GMO's

I had heard the term GMO, which stands for genetically modified organism. I didn't know what that meant when I first started my food journey. When I found out, I was appalled, and I want to make sure you understand it so you know why you should steer clear of GMO food whenever possible.

GMOs are created in a laboratory using genetic modification techniques. This means that the food has been genetically altered so that the plant produces more and is also more bug-resistant. Much of the food we eat has been genetically modified, especially meat, corn, soy, corn starch, vegetable oils, and sugar beets. Most processed food contains at least one of these ingredients.

Why are GMOs bad? To start, no one knows the long-term consequences of eating GMOs. Scientists from the FDA warn of potential allergies, toxins, new diseases, cancers, and nutritional problems and have urged long-term studies.

When I educated myself on GMOs, I realized that both GMO and processed foods were likely the main core issue with my digestive system.

Unfortunately, you can't avoid GMO products because they are everywhere, especially if you eat out as most food in restaurants will be made with GMOs. And as a busy mom and career woman, I like going out to eat!

But when I began to make my health the highest priority, I realized that to avoid consuming a high level of GMO foods, I had to cook. I decided to cook at least four to five days out of the seven-day week. Cooking was not that hard. I learned how to make meals in my slow cooker and pressure cooker—something I still do today, and I love it.

Those two or three days I didn't cook, I allowed the kids to order whatever they wanted. But here was the difference: I made sure it was something healthy and from an organic restaurant. You would be surprised to learn that the majority of your local small restaurants cook organic and healthy dishes.

How can you protect yourself from consuming GMO's? Eat organic as much as possible and avoid corn, soy, canola, sugar beets, high fructose corn syrup, maltodextrin, and soy protein which, again will be on the label of most processed food.

Eating Organic and from Local Farmers

Now that eating genetically modified organisms (GMOs) was no longer in my vocabulary, my next task was to find fresh local grown fruits and vegetables. It's not that I became obsessed with searching for non-GMOs items all the time. But I did make a conscious effort to choose the healthiest food I could. I owed it to myself and family.

After careful research, I discovered Community Supported Agriculture (CSA), a program that allows local people access to high quality, fresh produce from their local farmer. These farms use non-GMOs to grow their produce and fruits.

Similar to my local meat market, CSA provides an opportunity to purchase a "share" of vegetables and fruits from my local farmer. I suggest you google Community Supported Agriculture to find your local CSA.

My health coach also taught me the necessity of eating organic. Organic food is healthier. Organic fruits and vegetables are grown without dangerous pesticides and herbicides that are used on most fruits and vegetables. These dangerous chemicals are also sprayed on the feed given to chickens, cows, pigs, and sheep (as I noted above)—our main sources of protein.

Pesticides and herbicides have been proven to disrupt hormone production throughout our endocrine system. This is why they are not okay on an anti-inflammatory diet. You want foods that will help your endocrine system to work more efficiently—not the opposite.

Organic is basically like the food our great-great grandparents grew in their gardens. And research has found organic to taste better.

Once I started buying organic food, I noticed a huge change in my taste buds and digestive system. For instance, I never really enjoyed eating apples because they tasted like wax. When I purchased organic apples, it didn't have the waxy taste, and it was much juicier.

Of course, it's not always easy to eat only organic. When you can't, at least try to eat food with the least amount of pesticides. According to the Environmental Working Group, the foods below are the ones with the most amount of pesticides and should be replaced by organic sources. They are ordered from most pesticides used to least used.

Dirty Dozen

1. Strawberries
2. Spinach
3. Nectarines
4. Apples
5. Grapes
6. Peaches
7. Cherries
8. Pears
9. Tomatoes
10. Celery
11. Potatoes
12. Sweet Bell Peppers and Hot Peppers

Conversely, here are the "Clean 14" foods that aren't as heavily doused with pesticides and herbicides:

1. Avocados
2. Pineapples
3. Cabbage
4. Onions
5. Sweet peas frozen
6. Papayas
7. Asparagus
8. Mangos
9. Eggplant
10. Honeydew Melon
11. Kiwi
12. Cantaloupe
13. Cauliflower
14. Broccoli

However, it is best to buy organic when possible because even the "Clean 14" are sprayed with some pesticides and herbicides.

Eating Seasonally

To thrive, your body must adjust to changes in the weather.

As the winter starts approaching, my body starts changing. Once I started using food as medicine, I noticed that when it got cold, my body was craving more protein and carbs. It didn't matter how many fruits and vegetables I ate, my body still wanted more protein and carbs.

The colder it gets, the more my body craves soup. Because of my nutrition and health classes, when this first happened, I didn't freak out because I knew this was a normal change to the seasons. In the winter, I crave proteins, carbs, and grounding foods like soup because it helps me find balance. I don't have the feeling of constant hunger when I have a hearty bowl of soup. I love the comfort of the hot soup on a cold winter's day. It gives me a sense of peace.

Because this has been going on for many years now, I have become skillful in making soups: vegetable soup, lentil soup, and tomato soup but especially chicken noodle soup, my favorite soup. Called the "Jewish penicillin," chicken soup is truly full of ingredients to help support the immune system. That's why it helps keep those colds at bay in the winter.

I make mine with fresh diced carrots, celery, sweet onions, green onions, garlic, ginger, green pepper, yellow pepper, and red pepper. My spices are thyme, pepper, oregano, tarragon, cayenne pepper, cumin, and chicken bouillon.

I purchase my chicken breast from the local butcher. I also ask for the chicken back and bones which have the most minerals and make a very good broth. No matter what ingredients you use, season your chicken well and add a tablespoon of raw apple cider vinegar to help pull out the minerals from the chicken bones.

Place everything in the slow cooker. Add water until it covers the chicken. I fill the slow cooker half way because I love to drink the broth. (I have more to say on slow cookers in the next chapter.) You can decide how much water to add. Just make sure you cover everything enough to have soup. Slow cook for seven to eight hours on low. Come home from work. Serve. Feel cozy and well-cared for!

Superfoods

In my quest to find foods that heal, I also learned about superfoods. These are foods that give your body the extra added boost it needs for nutrition and that provide support for your microbiome system, which is your gut flora.

Many believe a poor microbiome system is at the heart of most disease. I'll talk more about this in a later chapter when I talk about the need to eat fermented foods.

There is a long list of superfoods to eat to build your nutrition. I enjoy blueberries, blackberries, honey, seaweed, chlorella, Maca, beans, kale, and ginger and feel that these foods help my digestive system work better and also provide stability for my thyroid.

Which ones you choose to eat all depends on what works for and tastes good to you. I advise everyone to experiment with different superfoods to gain an understanding of how it works for their body.

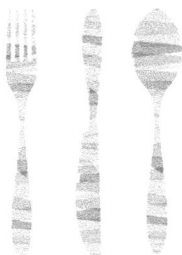

CHAPTER SEVEN

Mindful Eating

I HAVE TO ADMIT, CHANGING TO A HEALTHY WAY OF LIVING WAS HARD FOR me. I had been eating poorly my whole life, though I didn't know it and this style of cooking was not natural in my life. It was a struggle, and I didn't always stick to how my health coach has taught me to eat.

Also, I was the coupon queen, and my pantry was full of processed food purchased on a dime. In my mind, we were eating healthy because I was cooking more and eating out less. *That* was my definition of healthy! Little wonder that I was still struggling with digestive problems and occasional headaches.

Changing Mindset

So, what made me succeed? My belief in God and understanding that eating healthy is a mindset. In order to change your diet, you have to want to change the way you view food because food requires a relationship.

If you don't develop a relationship with food and understand how it affects your body and what works for you, you will continue to struggle with your food choices and ignore the signs of your body rejecting the food.

When I eat something, my body immediately tells me the food or dish wasn't good for me by giving me a headache, nausea, or reflux. I take note of the signs and try to find ways to improve the dish or eliminate it from my vocabulary.

Food should be your therapy; it should make you feel good not for a moment but for a lifetime. It should have no side effects or leave you disappointed about your decision. It should not show up negatively in your life. It should provide you joy, happiness, and give you a sense of pride. If it does leave you disappointed, you always have the opportunity to make it right by getting back to eating what your body needs for health—even with the next meal!

I started to explore the world of food via online search engines, health conferences, and books and learned many ways I could change my cooking. I have done it all from becoming a vegan, vegetarian, and pescatarian. (*Pesca* is fish in Latin/Italian, so that means I was a fish eater.)

Becoming Vegetarian

After my thyroid was removed, I was at a point in my life where food was the enemy. I couldn't keep anything in my stomach without feeling nauseous or vomiting. I decided to quit food. Of course, I couldn't quit food, so I decided to do a one week detox and only eat fruits and vegetables. The one week detox lasted a year, and I became a vegetarian.

Once I eliminated meat from my diet, I began to feel my body change for the better. This likely happened because meat is hard to digest and takes a long-time to go through the system—as long as four days. Fruits and vegetables digest quickly, and with all my digestive issues, I needed "quick exit" foods.

Also, processed meat has toxins, hormones, antibiotics, and other harmful substances. The worst offenders are cold cuts, bacon, sausages, hot dogs, and barbecued meat.

The only way to avoid eating these bad substances is to eat free range, organic and preferably grass-fed beef, eggs, and poultry. But free range, organic meat is very expensive—a steak for dinner might cost you $20. So, all in all, I decided it best to stop eating meat altogether—at least for a while.

Learning to Eat Veggies

Of course, to become a vegetarian I had to eat a lot of veggies and fruits. At first, this was hard as I never was a vegetable lover and my vocabulary for fruit ended at strawberries. The key to me loving vegetables and fruits was training my taste buds with a tongue cleaner.

I didn't stay a vegetarian because my body wanted meat. I learned that fish was a wonderful source of protein. I tried it and my body loved it. I could feel the energy my body got from the fish, so I became a pescatarian.

Meat vs. Vegetarian

I also noticed my body desired meat in the winter time because it was a grounding food for my body, giving it the support it needed to feel complete.

While I had become vegetarian and then later pescatarian, I had always missed eating meat. But now I learned that I could eat meat again *if* it was organic locally produced meat and I didn't eat too much of it. (I also know people who do well with grass fed/grass finished beef. This means the cow has eaten grass its whole life. It didn't go to the feed lot and get fattened up on corn before it was butchered).

I started searching for a local farmer who had good beef. To my surprise, I found several local farmers that use organic and non-antibiotic ways to raise their animals. And….my local meat market offered meat packages. For example, you can get a $40, $50, $60 package full of good healthy meat. I spent around $150 to $200 a month on meat for the whole family.

I didn't start eating a steak for dinner. Not only would that have been expensive but it also would have exacerbated my gastric reflex—bringing my food up is the worse experience for me. I hate it!

So when I first started introducing meat back into my life, I made it more of a condiment than the main course. Using this method worked great, and it helped me realize I didn't need meat all the time. I now eat meat maybe two or three days a month, and I never eat more than four ounces at a time—most of the time it's two ounces or less.

In the summertime, I don't eat meat because it makes me feel weighed down, and that's when I really feel it not digesting well.

My body adjusts to the seasons, and it works well for me. In the winter, I eat my soup because it grounds me. In the summer, I need light cooling foods like salads, fruits, raw veggies, and fish. My body is happy, and I'm thriving because of it.

Slow Cooker

One way of cooking that helped me make the change to a new, healthier way of eating was to cook with a slow cooker. I've already given you my chicken soup recipe. It can't be done unless you have a slow cooker.

If you don't know how to cook, I suggest you start with this method. It is one of the most underrated kitchen items. Rather than slave over a pot for hours, a slow cooker allows you to return five, six, eight, even ten hours later to a cooked meal of mainly fresh ingredients.

Because it is cooked at a low temperature for a long time, the food retains much of its nutrition-rich, natural juices from vegetables and meats. The internet is a great start to finding recipes for cooking with a slow cooker. I enjoy the videos. (Since I have a hard time focusing, watching a video is much easier for me. It may be for you as well.)

Prepacking

If you lead a busy life like me, I suggest pre-packing your slow cooker meals by placing the ingredients in a plastic bag in the freezer. When it is time to start cooking, you place it (frozen or thawed) in the slow cooker and turn it on! If you go online, you will see people pre-packing for a month. I suggest you start with a few days a week or a week-long prepackage meal.

Changing the way you eat takes time. It requires discipline because you can't just "grab something quick." Meals need to be planned and you need to add cooking into your daily routine. It's what works for you, like me being a pescatarian most of the time but eating meat sparingly a few times a month, or my editor who eats mostly veggies and no more than 8 ounces of meat a day (with red meat at most twice a week).

Your relationship to food is important. Food plays a huge role in our lives. Our comfort food comes with wonderful memories. Foods that have made us sick in the past are foods we generally shun. But the most important thing you can remember about food is that if you're eating food that your body can use for energy, then it is some of the most powerful medicine available on the planet.

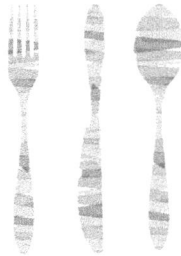

CHAPTER EIGHT

Good Health Routines

THE JOURNEY TOWARDS GOOD HEALTH IS NOT A NICE LINEAR ONE. IT TAKES twists and turns, and you find that what worked for you for a while doesn't work so well in the present moment. So you need to learn to be flexible and listen to what your body is telling you.

I also know that there are some really important routines that play into good health. I adopted my routines years ago and have kept them in because they continue to support my body and give me that energy and verve for life that I've come to not only enjoy but count on as my life gets busier helping others through their own health issues.

Healing the Gut

After I became a vegetarian, I was on the road to living my best life. But I was still concerned about repairing my gut. I was digesting food better, but it wasn't always the best. That's when I learned about the microbiome.

Let me explain. Microbes are found in your gut and are essential to how well you digest your food. If you don't eat healthy foods to help populate your gut with bacteria-fighting microbes, your microbes start to die off.

When this happens, you get a leaky gut. Leaky gut means you have intestinal permeability. Bad substances leak out of the lining of the small intestine and into the bloodstream and toxins flood your body. When toxins flood your body, you develop inflammation. (See how that's all connected?)

This is what happened to me and caused so many digestive issues. The good news is you can save your microbes by eating healthy fruits, vegetables, and fermented foods! Yes!

Fermented Foods

Fermented foods have been around for years, and different countries have a different way of fermenting their food. For example, Korea has Kimchi, and China has Kombucha. Kombucha is my favorite fermented beverage.

I do not ferment my food because it can be dangerous if you don't ferment it properly. I purchase my fermented food from the local organic supermarket.

Recently, I noticed more fermented foods and beverages in my local grocery store; for example, they have a large section of Kombucha, Kavita, Kefir, and yogurt. Yes, certain yogurt is fermented.

I would advise you do your research and experiment with different fermented foods and beverages to see which one works for you. A great book to read on this subject is *The Lose Your Belly Diet* by Dr. Travis Stork, M.D. You know him from the T.V. show The Doctors.

The fermentation process promotes the growth of the healthy bacteria your gut needs to function properly. When you eat that healthy bacteria, it gets in your gut, makes the right changes, and then your digestion works better. It's why you'll see "live cultures" on some yogurt containers. These live cultures are the good bacteria. Your body will tell you when it's had enough. You'll get diarrhea if you eat too much. If you suffer from constipation, probiotics (another way of saying the good bacteria), help your bowels move. That's what you want—good, healthy, daily elimination.

So Many Changes

Once I introduced my body to pre-probiotics (super fruits), fermented foods/beverages, CSA (Community Supported Agriculture) and the local meat market, it started to heal itself. I started feeling better, healthier, and more alive than ever before.

My gym routine was more meaningful because I started to see a more consistent progression in my body. Remember, I was always slim, but I didn't look healthy because my weight would fluctuate because of my thyroid and digestive system.

I was no longer exhausted, and I didn't suffer from migraines.

Eventually, my appetite started to grow, and I was eating more and feeling complete. Thanksgiving came around, and the family decided to have it at my house. I was excited because it was an opportunity to show my family my new lifestyle. Unfortunately, my aunt wouldn't hear of it! She cooked all the food at her house except the turkey.

I didn't get upset because I was happy to be with my family. I did purchase an organic turkey from my local CSA.

The next month, my aunt became ill. She went to the emergency room on Friday and passed away the next week on Thursday. Her death was sudden, and hit the family hard because she was just with us for Thanksgiving.

She had complained about her gastric reflux, and we didn't think anything of it because she suffered from gastric reflux for years. She even said, "I had this before, and it will eventually go away." Passing away a few months later was a surprise. The doctors believe she had pancreatic cancer which is almost always fatal. The cause is hard to diagnose, but my theory is it was from the gastric reflux.

I miss my aunt, just as I miss my mother terribly. But all in all, my life is hugely happier and more fulfilling because I am not continuing to eat the way I did growing up.

The Importance of Water

Our bodies are made up mostly of water—up to 60%! If you're not drinking enough water, your body doesn't function well. Your body can't flush the toxins and that causes problems in your kidneys. Water is a very important component to digestion, and is also vital to your brain functioning well.

The general rule is to drink eight, eight-ounce glasses of water a day. Some nutritionists and doctors recommend you sip water all day long. How you consume it is again dependent on how it makes you feel.

The Best Water to Drink

Listen, if you ask me there is no "best" water. Just drink water! I used to buy bottled water, but then I read about the chemicals from the plastic seeping into the water, as well as the effects that the increasing number of bottles is having on the environment. I decided to use tap water that is filtered in a container that does not have any BPA (bisphernol A). This is a chemical used in a lot of plastics and in the lining of many tin cans, and it has been shown to disrupt hormone balances, making a body more estrogenic (even in men), which then disrupts all sorts of other hormonal reactions. We don't want that to happen!

Having a filter is very important because some places in the world have good purification systems, while others leave traces of chlorination by-products, lead, and sometimes bacteria. Research your area and educate yourself on where your water is coming from. My sister has a fresh water spring right up to the road from her house. I'm so jealous. Can you believe she does not take advantage of it?

If you find yourself exhausted, sleepy, bloated, backaches, headaches, digestive problem, or out of whack, drink more water because you could be dehydrated.

Also, don't think that drinking soda, energy drinks, tea, or coffee will hydrate you. I love coffee, but I also know coffee is a dehydrating drink. Yes, these are our favorite beverages, and they do contain water, but they also contain items that dehydrate you.

The best way to identify your water need is to measure your age, diet, activity, health, and climate. (And don't get sidetracked by reports that say drinking too much water can cause a mineral imbalance and lack of sleep. We're talking gallons here, so don't use that as an excuse not to drink plenty of water!).

These are my experiences with water, and some people might think differently. The bottom line is drink water!

Tongue Cleaner

A tongue cleaner scrapes the bacteria off of your tongue. It's a great way to help with changing your taste buds because it cleans all toxic mucus that can block your taste for the food. And it has other great healthy benefits like preventing toxins from getting into your body from the residue on your tongue, preventing bad breath, and improving gum health.

Cleaning my tongue allowed me to taste the natural nutrients food had to offer. Think about it, if you never cleaned your tongue, imagine how much residue would be on it? It reminds me of someone who never vacuums their carpet. When you decide to vacuum, the container is full of dirt. What about that cheese burger you had last month or the rib sauce you can still taste from a year ago?

Seriously, a tongue cleaner is a great way to clean your mouth and have a fresh start each day for the taste of life.

Pulling Oil

Pulling oil has been gaining in popularity recently. It comes from Ayurveda medicine (a traditional Indian system of health). I "pull oil" because it has wonderful healthy benefits. It helps control plaque build-up and gingivitis. It also kills microorganisms that cause bad breath. It moistens the mouth, lips, and throat.

The antibacterial properties of oil pull out bacteria and fungus, alleviating inflammation, congestion, and even allergies. Oil pulling is even said to relieve stomach issues such as ulcers and improve kidney function.

While some of these benefits are not proven by actual study, I know that I feel a lot better when I do it.

This is how you pull oil:

❖ Take one tablespoon oil and swish it around your mouth for twenty minutes and spit it out. You can use coconut oil, sesame oil, or sunflower oil. It is best to use pure organic oil. When you're ready to spit it out, make sure you do so in the garbage. The contaminated oil can clog your pipes.

❖ When you're done pulling, rinse your mouth out with salt water or water mixed with a little apple cider vinegar. This is to make sure all the oil is out of your mouth.

❖ Next, brush your teeth well to kill any bacteria left over.

❖ You can pull oil any time of the day, but it is best to pull oil in the morning.

❖ It is best to start off small; I could only do it for two-to-three minutes when I first did it. Eventually, you will move up to twenty minutes. It took me some time, but I made it to twenty minutes after a few months of consistently pulling oil.

❖ DO NOT SWALLOW the oil. If you are struggling with it in your mouth, you have too much. A little goes a long way.

I learned that you can use any of the above oils to fight bacteria and gain healthy benefits; however, coconut oil is best to use. It has the added benefit of lauric acid, which is well-known for its anti-microbial agents making it more effective. Also, a recent study found that coconut oil may help prevent tooth decay.

Killing the Sugar Addiction

Because my mother had put sugar into all her cooking, I was, like the rest of the nation, addicted to sugar. She also always kept a bottle of soda pop in the house. We rarely had water or juice in the house. All this sugar only added to my symptoms. Of course, for me, the problem wasn't weight gain as it is for most people, but inflammation was all through my body.

To help me stop eating processed, refined sugar, I researched alternatives and started using maple sugar, molasses, and honey. If I decided to use sugar, I chose raw sugar which I learned about during a safari trip to the Dominican Republic.

In the Dominican Republic, I was introduced to coffee bean and raw sugar. It was the best coffee I ever tasted, and it only required a teaspoon of raw sugar. I had no clue it was sugar because it was brown. After talking to the natives, they explained it was raw sugar and that, unlike refined sugar which has no added nutrients, raw sugar has a small number of nutrients.

To me, coffee with raw sugar is so delicious, and I admit, I love it and drink it every day.

However, I know that this is something that will need to be removed from my diet. Why do I have to give up coffee? Coffee is a stimulant and, because of my thyroid, I suffer from anxiety. The caffeine doesn't help. So, I have had to try and at least cut back on drinking coffee and replacing it with alternatives like barley teas that taste like coffee.

However, sugar is an entirely different story. Did you know that sugar has fifty-six different types or names? I was in disbelief when I read this in a blog. The next time you read a label, make sure you check for these names. Please keep in mind this list could have changed:

1. High-Fructose Corn Syrup (HFCS)
2. Agave Nectar
3. Beet sugar
4. Blackstrap molasses
5. Brown sugar
6. Buttered syrup
7. Cane juice crystals
8. Cane sugar
9. Caramel
10. Carob Syrup
11. Castor sugar
12. Coconut sugar
13. Confectioner's sugar (powdered sugar)
14. Date sugar
15. Demerara sugar
16. Evaporated cane juice
17. Florida Crystals
18. Fruit juice
19. Fruit juice concentrate
20. Golden sugar
21. Golden syrup
22. Grape sugar
23. Honey
24. Icing sugar
25. Invert sugar
26. Maple syrup
27. Molasses
28. Muscovado sugar
29. Panela sugar
30. Raw sugar
31. Refiner's syrup
32. Sorghum syrup
33. Sucanat
34. Treacle sugar
35. Turbinado sugar
36. Yellow sugar
37. Barley malt
38. Brown rice syrup
39. Corn syrup
40. Corn syrup solids
41. Dextrin
42. Dextrose
43. Diastatic malt
44. Ethyl maltol
45. Glucose
46. Glucose solids
47. Lactose
48. Malt syrup
49. Maltodextrin
50. Maltose
51. Rice syrup
52. Crystalline Fructose

Sugar is everywhere and pretty much in everything. It makes things taste good, which means you buy more of the food being offered. But it wreaks havoc on a body, so the less you can eat it, the better.

It may be really hard to give it up. Your body craves it for about a week to two weeks after you stop using it. But after a while, you don't want it. You don't like how it makes you feel, and things become much tastier and even sweeter naturally when you don't use sugar. Honestly, the best sugar is naturally found in our fruits.

Spices

One of the key discoveries in helping me switch to a healthier way of eating was discovering seasoning. Having been raised on seasoning salt and paprika for everything, and a dash of sugar for sweetness, I underestimated the power of fresh herbs and spices. Herbs and spices are two different things, and I love them both.

They both provide the tasteful joy you need in your food. Herbs are the leafy part of a plant and spices come from the rest of the plant, like the fruit, seeds, root, bark, kernel, stem, etc.

You can grind, crush, or make your herbs and spices into a paste. However you prepare them, they make your food delicious.

This was an important discovery, but one that took a while for me to switch to. I was used to the rich taste of food laden with fat, sugar, and salt. At first the healthy food I was now eating was too dull. To make food more palatable, I put sugar and salt on everything. But masking the food with sugar and salt was no better than eating the unhealthy way.

I had to do my research. I found different dishes to cook and learned to experiment with spices to help retrain my taste buds. My experimenting helped me learn the benefits of natural spices for seasoning instead of pouring on the unhealthy salt. My children didn't know the difference, and my household was slowly adjusting to not putting salt on everything. Over time, I began to notice that I didn't need salt and was able to limit it in my diet.

It took a while, but it got a lot easier when eventually I became vegetarian. Exploring different ways to create seasoning was great fun and became my hobby.

My favorite mix that I call my "magical spice" is garlic, rosemary, thyme, tarragon, onion, and cayenne pepper.

I have to single out ginger for a moment. I love it. I use ginger in almost everything. I love especially making ginger tea. Ginger provides the body with everything from helping the digestive system to nausea and is one of nature's biggest anti-inflammatories. I found it helped to relieve inflammation and boost my immunity.

Try blending ginger with fresh lemon juice and water. It tastes delicious, and the health benefits will send your digestive system into a detox. I suggest you try the ginger candy from the health food store. I love it!

All in all, my dishes turned into delicious family meals, and my secret was in the spices. One of my favorites, and a quick dish, is Zucchini Pasta. You cut the zucchini into cubes and pour a teaspoon of extra virgin olive oil in a cast iron pan.

Once hot, add the zucchini and onions. Once the zucchini starts to get soft add green peppers, red peppers, garlic, and spices (garlic powder, cayenne, onion power, basil, tarragon, and thyme). Place fresh tomatoes in a blender with extra virgin olive and blend until almost liquid. I like to taste the chunks of tomatoes so I don't blend it too much. Pour the juice from the blender in the pan and simmer for fifteen minutes! Serve over pasta (preferably rice pasta) or brown rice.

Teas

Along with eating healthy food, I learned the enormous health benefit of teas. I find them calming and rejuvenating.

Tea provides healthy fluids to your body and heart. Studies have shown tea can have a positive effect on diet, contains antioxidants, a great substitute for coffee, and prevents some diseases.

In place of buying teabags, I prefer natural tea leaves, and I grow my peppermint tea and lemon balm tea.

Peppermint tea gives me mental awareness to help me focus on the daily task and relieves my headaches. It also has anti-inflammatory proprieties that help with the *Erythema Nodosum* and thyroid flares that I still occasionally experience.

Lemon balm helps me sleep at night. It is great also for digestive problems, menstrual cramps, headaches, etc. I have also heard it is great for children with ADHD. It helps me relax and clear my mind because it supports my thyroid disease.

I have an entire collection of teas that provide similar benefits, and my family knows about this. For this reason, I often receive a natural tea collection for my birthday, Christmas, or holiday. My niece is the best at giving me tea gifts because she purchases my tea collection from a place in Pittsburg that has all natural tea leaves grown there.

I suggest finding a quiet place to reflect on your day and drink a cup of tea to help you absorb the great qualities of your life.

Essential Oils

As I began to incorporate healing modalities, my family and friends noticed…I would even say I made their head "spin" a little. One thing that I insisted that everyone try was the use of essential oils. It's called "aromatherapy."

Aromatherapy is the use of essential oils to awake the senses in your body, both by breathing in the healing components of the oils and through absorption directly onto your skin.

Different oils have different effects. Some like lavender and rose are calming, while others like lemon and peppermint are alerting, while others like eucalyptus have direct healing properties for illness. People will be drawn to which scents they choose for their own needs.

I first discovered aromatherapy when a friend who would post all of these essential oils on Facebook and talked about how it provided so much relief in many different areas. I became curious and started to research essential oils.

The more I read about their healing powers, the more I wanted to try these oils on me. The local community college was offering a certification course on essential oil, and I decided to take the course.

It was amazing and taught me how to use these oils in healing and relaxing ways. I bought a diffuser and started using lavender oil to help me relax and sleep at night.

Lavender is the "universal oil" and the most popular and versatile of all essential oils. It's lightly sweet, and its fresh floral scent has proven effective in treating tension, depression, headaches, and insomnias, as well as PMS. I love the scent and use it daily, and it has provided me some relief to my ailments.

Using Essential Oils

Essential oils are expensive. If you diffuse them, you will typically use several dabs at a time that will last a few hours. If you put them directly on the skin, you only put on a few dabs as the oils have a powerful effect on the body and you can overload your system. If you mix the oils to make cream, you want to use a sparing amount at one time. You should be able to smell the scent but not strongly, as you would with perfume.

All-in-all, it's best to become educated on how to use essential oils as I did. I suggest you start off with the standard oils, for example, lavender, eucalyptus, and peppermint. Once you become comfortable and have done your research, you can venture out to ylang-ylang, citrus, sandalwood, and others.

Also, be careful about ingesting them. Though I have had people ask me about taking essential oils by mouth. I have tried ingesting essential oils, but only from a safe, well-known company. Before you ingest them, remember, essential oils are chemicals. Whenever you're using chemicals you should be cautious and get educated on the effects it will have on your body. Once you drink these oils, the effect it has on your body is different from the effect it has when they are applied topically.

If you do wish to try ingesting them, do your research and find out which oils are safe to ingest and the quantity.

Essential Oils and Skin

Once I saw the power of "aromatherapy" or the use of essential oils for healing, the next step was using essential oils in my skin care.

I was born with sensitive, dry skin. My skin would bruise easily, and I would often have fine little bumps or red blotches on my body. Since I was suffering from *Erythema Nodosum*, it would leave these huge bruises on my legs. One summer, I refused to wear shorts because of the bruises.

I purchased organic Shea Butter, Coconut Oil, and essential oils and started making my body cream. I made creams with lavender, frankincense, rose, and other calming oils to help me sleep at night.

Then I started making creams with citrus, peppermint, eucalyptus, and other waking oils to help me wake up and be refreshed for the day.

All of my body creams started to provide me with more focus during the day and also provided a calming effect at night. They were especially great while doing yoga—my main form of exercise that I will discuss in the next chapter—because they helped give me added strength.

I began to wonder. If these are good chemicals having direct contact with your internal organs, image what harmful chemicals are doing to your internal organs and circulation. It made me aware of the chemicals around me and the skin-to-touch contact.

Of course, I was aware that it's impossible to avoid all contact with toxins and bacteria. You don't want to avoid bad things, especially bacteria, altogether because then your body can't build up your immune system to fight off the bad stuff. Let me explain. If you avoid bad chemicals and bacteria all the time, your body goes on vacation. It stops working on building up the strength to ward off the bad things you come in contact with in life.

When the time does come for the body to fight, it's not ready because it has been on vacation. This allows you to become susceptible to sickness, etc.

Bottom line—I am mindful of the things I interact with daily. I have taken the time to educate myself on what is good and not good for a body, then tried it on me. If something doesn't work for me, then I don't continue doing it just because someone said "this works." I have made a point of making wise choices about my food and the chemicals I put in and on my body, and I urge you to do the same.

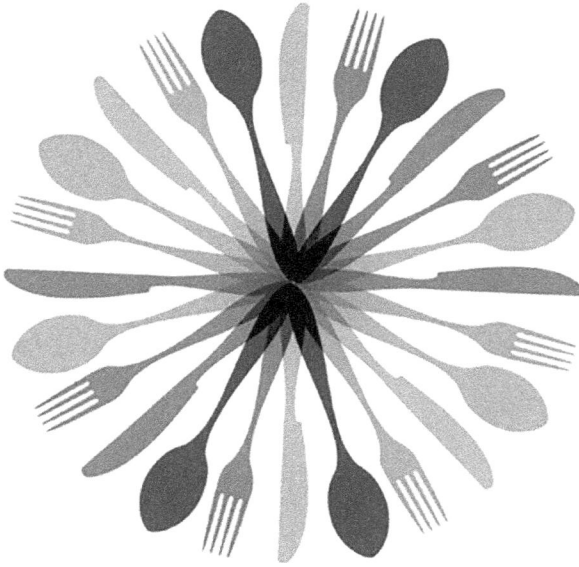

PART FOUR

Spiritual Growth

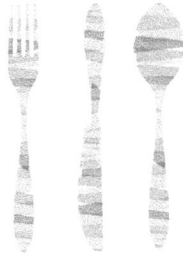

CHAPTER NINE

Finding Strength in a Spiritual Path

IN THE BEGINNING OF THE BOOK I TALKED ABOUT BALANCE—WHAT IT means and how it's something that we're constantly striving for. I have also talked quite a bit about the importance of maintaining hormonal balance, primarily by changing your mindset about the way you eat first, and the being mindful all the time of what's going into your mouth.

Balance, however, doesn't mean that everything stays the same. Balance is something you work on creating every day. Some days are more unbalanced than others, obviously, and when that happens, it's okay to hit the "reset" button. Start over. Figure out what's out and move forward from there.

I have always believed in God and the power a supreme being brings into our lives.

But I was also living the way most everyone else does in America—in a sort of *carpe diem*, live for the day, kind of way. The goiter in my throat was not going away. I wasn't well because I had all the symptoms of hyper thyroid. But at that time in my life, I felt it was more important that I care for my sons and work on advancing my career.

As I related before, I knew that I needed to do something about the growing bulge in my throat. But right before my mother was diagnosed with cancer—there were two other life-changing events that really made me stop and look at how I was living my life not just physically, but spiritually. Where was my life's journey really taking me?

My Son's Heart Condition

The first happened when my wonderful seventeen-year old son was rushed to the hospital because he was dying. His heart wasn't working. To make matters worse, he wasn't in Baltimore, where we lived. He had gone to Atlanta for the summer to work for my cousin who owned her own business.

In the weeks leading up to his hospitalization, we were all excited because my first-born child was exploring the world of work. He had just received his driving licenses a year earlier, so getting around Atlanta was going to be a breeze.

Personally I welcomed the break because like any seventeen-year-old boy, he was at the crossroads of life and we often disagreed on everything from school, cleaning his room, dinner, and of course what he was wearing.

One day shortly after he arrived in Atlanta, I received a phone call from my uncle that my son wasn't feeling well, and they were taking him to the doctor. The doctor diagnosed him with an upset stomach and sent him home. My son's condition started to worsen but he refused to go back to the doctor.

Within a week, he was in my cousin's room vomiting and having stomach pains but still refusing to go the doctor. My family called me, and I screamed at him from the top of my lungs to go the hospital. He went to the doctor and they sent him home again.

The next night he was rushed to the hospital.

He had myocarditis. Myocarditis is inflammation of the heart muscle. The cause is unknown. The prognosis is chronic heart failure which means long-term complication.

When my son left for Atlanta, he looked like a healthy seventeen-year-old child who played several sports throughout his life. Now, my beautiful child was fighting for his life on an ECMO (extracorporeal membrane oxygenation) machine, a machine that takes over the work of the heart and lungs. It gives a very sick body the ability to rest and hopefully recover.

Describing what I went through is difficult because of the uncontrollable emotions and feelings that ran through my mind. My son never had any major-medical concerns to make us think he would need a heart transplant. He played basketball and football from age six to seventeen-years old.

The first hospital wasn't equipped to assist him, so he was rushed to Children's Hospital in Atlanta. When my son arrived in the emergency room, the doctors started talking to him about his condition, and that's when he went into cardiac arrest.

My cousin couldn't ride in the ambulance, so she drove behind it. When she walked through the door, she saw doctors surrounding my son and machines trying to bring him back to life. She dropped in the middle of the emergency room floor with her hands in the air crying out to God to please save her cousin.

My aunt called me around 1:00 a.m. to tell me that my son was in the hospital.

I immediately called my mother, sister, and aunt we arranged for me to take the next flight to Atlanta. After hanging up the phone with my family I called my pray warrior and best friend, we started to pray. We prayed all night and into the early morning.

I knew then that God would not conceal my son's death from me, so therefore he would not take my son. It was an attack of the enemy, and I was going to pray until things changed. It was during this time that I learned the meaning of warfare prayer.

When I arrived at the airport, my aunt called to give me an update. They had gotten him stable and were placing him on the ECMO machine. They needed my agreement to bill my insurance.

The nurses also indicated they needed to wake him up from sedation for less than a minute before placing him on the ECMO. I agreed to everything.

My cousin came back on the phone, and I told her to give the phone to the chaplain who was with my son. I told the priest to stay with my son and read Psalm 118:7 continually out loud to him until I arrived: "I will not die but live, and will proclaim what the LORD has done."

I hung up the phone and went into a corner at the airport, sat on the floor, called my girlfriend, and we prayed until it was time to board the plane. I prayed against everything that was attacking my son. I could feel the presence of calmness on the plane, and I knew my son was going to be healed.

God gave me a sense of peace. I could feel Matthew 10:26: "So do not be afraid of them, for there is nothing concealed that will not be disclosed, or hidden that will not be made known."

My uncle picked me up from the airport and took me straight to the hospital. I arrived at the airport in the afternoon, hugged and kissed my family, grabbed my prayer cloth and anointing oil, and went to my son.

When I walked in the room, my son was surrounded by several machines, and tubes were everywhere. His bed was raised almost above our heads and there were tubes in his mouth, tubes in his neck, tubes in his arms, tubes in his groin area. It felt like someone punched me in my stomach and took the breath out of me. My head was swimming in confusion and panic and the very person that gave me life to live was fighting for his life. I started praying over the machines with the oil and placed the prayer cloth across his waist.

After a week, my son was taken off the ECMO machine. His heart couldn't handle the stress of beating on its own, so they gave him a pacemaker, but they didn't release him from the hospital to go home. He first had to go to a rehabilitation hospital.

I never left my son. I stayed in his room praying. The hospital had dorm-like rooms as sleeping areas for parents, so I stayed in the dorm room. Day and night, I was in the room with my son praying and talking to him about everything. I played Christian music in the room and read stories and scriptures to him.

For a week, I went without eating. Thanks to the Ronald McDonald house, my husband and I were able to stay there. The program was amazing. They provided food and a full kitchen for you to cook. I had no energy to cook, but I did enjoy eating the food that was donated.

It was a blessing to come to the room after being at the hospital all day and seeing food available to eat. I thought it would be McDonalds every day, but it wasn't McDonalds; restaurants donated meals to the families.

After several months, my son required a heart transplant. This was a very serious operation. He survived, and I know it was because he was surrounded by constant prayer. I have always given the praise and glory to God for his survival.

I was relieved that my son was going to live—even though it meant a lifetime of medication and advanced health-care. But my health deteriorated further because I was not taking care of my body, at all.

Of course, I had long cancelled my goiter surgery. If I hadn't been living a life in prayer, I'm sure the stress of watching my son constantly fight for his life would have done me in. I didn't know how truly ill I was. I figured out later that my whole entire endocrine system was completely out of whack, and it was only because I was praying so hard for my son that I'm sure God spared me.

It was a realization I would come to later, and it would change my whole outlook on what balance really means. It's not just a balanced body, or even a balance between the body and mind, but a balance between our bodies and our spiritual selves that matter.

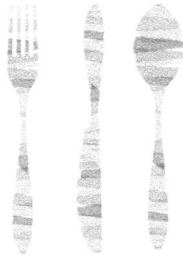

CHAPTER TEN

Letting Faith Guide Me

AFTER RETURNING HOME WITH MY SON, MY MOTHER BECAME SICK. THAT'S when she refused to go to the doctor until I went to mine to take care of my goiter. I had it removed, she passed away, and I finally had to take a hard look at how I was living.

I was taking the lessons to heart that my health coach had taught me. But in spite of eating better, I felt something was not right in my life. I was missing out on something.

I was very good at this point of suppressing the feeling of "not enough"— me not being "enough": a good enough mother, wife, or employee—because everyone around me kept telling me to appreciate the "enough" in my life. My mother and aunt taught me that you "go to work every day, have good health insurance, and save for retirement." So that is how I had lived my life. But it no longer was working.

Food and Mood

During the time, I spent with my health coach, she explained was that food is only one part of the equation. I must learn to lead a balanced lifestyle. She helped me understand that you could eat all the healthy foods in the world but if your life is out of balance, you would still be susceptible to sickness and disease.

Why? Food is only part of the nourishment to the body. If you are stressed out, your hormones are out of control and food will not sustain you. Being healthy is the ability to balance life and food, enjoyably and equally.

I started analyzing my life as a whole and realized how unhappy I was. My unhappiness was the cause of my lack of eating and my increase in weight loss. I know, I know.... if you are trying to lose weight, you are saying why is she complaining? Well, losing weight from stress is the unhealthiest way to lose weight because it reduces everything your body needs to sustain itself.

Ignoring My Authentic Self

I not only fault the doctors for my ignorance about what was best for my body and mind. I fault as well my inability to question rather than just accept. Though I had a few friends and family members who lived out their dreams and a few who are still working towards those dreams, I followed my mother and aunt's words and buried my dreams.

Such suppression of my dreams tormented my mind, body, and soul. It actually choked me. This is why I believe I got a goiter. I had silenced my dreams. Think about it; I didn't need medication. I had this large nodule growing in my throat. The goiter symbolized feeling choked in my life.

Why do we go through life suppressing the very thing that will bring us joy and freedom? Because it doesn't match society's view of happiness, or it's too scary and might destroy the "good thing" you have going on. And so we end up walking around with ailments and sickness.

And it's not just that we suppress joy and freedom. We also sometimes suppress pain. Yes, pain, the pain you are now experiencing in life.

But what if the thing you suppressed could bring you great things? If you knew, of course, you would change directions and run and leap towards your hopes and dreams. In hindsight, I can definitely say that instead of guessing, believe and move towards those hopes and dreams.

And this is what I was determined to do, starting with eating healthy. For healthy eating is more than a lifestyle, it is a way of being. It is who you are in the space that God has provided you and being okay with the journey you are taking.

I decided I was going to live life. Matthew 6:34 states, "Therefore do not worry about tomorrow, for tomorrow will worry about itself. Each day has enough trouble of its own." I impressed this verse on my heart, mind, body, and soul, so I would learn to live today, not tomorrow.

I started enjoying and being thankful for waking up in the morning, seeing my children's' beautiful faces, having a job that paid well, living in a beautiful home, driving a great car.

I started appreciating what I had instead of worrying about what I didn't have and worrying about losing it all. I had spent so much of my life being tuned into the "Lost Channel" (a channel that reminds you that you can lose everything at any minute, and you're not worthy of what you have) that I never accepted what I had. But I finally decided to tune into "Thankful Channel" (the channel that reminds you to be thankful of everything and open for more thankful blessings). That's when things really began to open up.

I was on my way to change. I knew the path would not be straight, but I prayed each day that God would lead me through the day. If I could just make it through the day, I was happy.

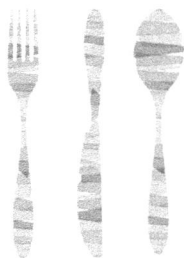

CHAPTER ELEVEN

Get Moving!

B RACED WITH MY NEW FAITH AND RENEWED SENSE OF MYSELF AS A DECENT person, I felt more courageous about facing all my many trials. It had been many years in the making. I had spent most of my life not taking care of myself, and the physical aftermath of living without my regulating thyroid gland caused all sorts of problems.

Then, I remembered everything I had to live for in life. My children are my strength. My oldest was a walking miracle of God's grace, and my youngest son was the voice of peace. I accepted that I had this condition, and I started to research a way to live with it, without medication if possible, and in a way that would allow me to live fully—not just physically but mentally and even spiritually.

Finding Yoga

The one thing one of the doctors told me after I had my thyroid removed that exercise helped balance hormones. I never enjoyed exercising because I didn't like to sweat. I had to find an activity that didn't require too much jumping around and, as I don't much like noise or yelling. I joined The YMCA and discovered yoga.

I decided that yoga would be the way I would tackle exercise, in much the same way my health coach had helped me get a handle on food. It would help me with the mind-body connection that I knew was missing.

Yoga requires flexibility and strength. You get into a pose, hold it, and then move to the next posture. But I was so out of shape and inflexible, I couldn't touch my toes and could barely do any of the many yoga postures. At first, I felt like I looked like a fool and was embarrassed half the time. I had a wonderful instructor who reminded us daily that in yoga, you never compare yourself to anyone else in class. Instead, we were to focus on the slow improvements we were making individually. Initially, that was hard for me to do.

Nevertheless, from the beginning, I loved it. I bought beginning yoga videos so I could practice at home every day of the week. On Saturday, I went to The Y for my classes.

After a few months, I was able to maintain my focus on yoga for at least thirty minutes and not worry about how bad I looked, or how much work I had to do, or on my digestive issues, or on the arthritic pain as I worked to hold a plank position (when you put your body in a push-up position but you hold it for a period of time). I was excited, and it was fun.

Yoga saved my life. Eventually, I became more flexible, my stiffness started to decrease, the function started to get better, balance started to improve, and yoga breathing helped decrease my anxiety and depression. That helped balance me mentally, which allowed me to find balance spiritually.

Yoga Breathing

During yoga practice, you are taught *Ujjai* (pronounced ooh-Jai-yee) breathing. You take a deep inhalation through your nose and exhale by constricting the back muscles in your throat. You will make a slight "dragon" or Darth Vader sound. If you open up your mouth and say "Haaaah" as if you're fogging up a mirror, you will know what the breath should sound like.

This simple breathing technique has a powerful influence on the body and mind. It balances the entire cardiorespiratory system, releases irritation, tension and frustration, and calms the mind and body. For me, learning to breathe correctly seemed to add years to my life and greatly decreased my stress level. It also relieved my headaches when nothing else would—and that alone was a life-saver!

Yoga Benefits

Many people take yoga for granted and think it is not a total body workout. But actually, yoga is a strenuous workout for the whole body, much more so than your average work out.

Yoga increases your flexibility around your joints and relieves tremendous stress and discomfort from your joints. During an hour to two-hour yoga practice, you take the joints in your body through a full range of motion to create, as the yogis say, more space in your body.

This helps to squeeze and soak areas of cartilage that aren't used much—to oil your joints so to speak. When your body is as tight and tense as mine was, it doesn't allow the blood to flow easily through the body and can cause some issues. The more flexible my body got, the less arthritic pain I felt. Yoga contains many weight bearing postures where you balance on one leg for instance, and these postures build bone strength. This helps osteoarthritis immensely because it helps strengthen the bones and cartilage.

Along with flexibility, yoga builds muscle strength, and I started to feel the pleasure of having actual muscles which gave me more body awareness. It felt different than lifting weights, which would only build strength.

And yoga builds a core. The core means the center of something, and in this case, it's the center of your body. If your core is strong, your body and your mind are strong and centered.

Yes, working your core helps you have beautiful tight abs, but the core is much more than abs. For one, when you strengthen your core, you also strengthen your digestive system. Because that is in the center of your body, you can also stabilize your organs, which helps stabilize blood and lymph flow, and, of course that helps the flow of hormones.

Yoga improved my core, helping my body feel more stable. It also taught me a lot about the core of our bodies.

Exercise

The more I learned about my thyroid disease, the more I learned about the importance of exercising more. I was doing yoga every week, but I needed more cardio.

If you are anything like me, you hate the gym, and you hate cardio. I am not the girl you see training for a marathon or walking to exercise. I dreaded having to do any type of cardio, but all roads lead to cardio exercise, and I knew I had to eventually go down that path.

Personal Trainer

The gym for me is a most confusing place because you never know if you are using the machines correctly. I certainly didn't want to look like a fool on the treadmill or lifting weights.

After a few failed attempts at the gym, I decided to hire a personal trainer. I found an inexpensive trainer fresh out of school. I learned it is best to find people who are starting a business or fresh out of the program because their rates are much lower. I'm a very frugal person, and I try to find a deal whenever possible. I was not about to spend a large sum of money on a trainer.

My trainer would come to my house once a week, and we would train. I would clear the basement out and make my area for exercising. I created motivational posters and placed them on the wall. I purchased a Bluetooth speaker, and my trainer would play different music to get me motivated. My exercise equipment only required an exercise mat, a jump rope, and a resistance band. Remember, I am very frugal.

It was great because I was able to explain my health condition and goals, and he created a workout plan around me achieving my goals that looked like this. I started with a thirty-second plank position, three sets of five lunges, exercises on the mat (sit-ups, etc.) and resistance bands to strengthen my overall body.

Resistance bands are a great exercise tool because you can perform many exercises with them and they enhance the conditioning. For example, you can do a front squat where you stand on the band with your feet hip-width apart, hold the band in each hand, squat, and pull the band up to your shoulders. It provides both cardio and weight training (but without the weights) because you are using your body's energy against itself. It's very effective.

Each resistance band has different levels of resistance. I suggest starting with the least resistance and working your way up to the different levels. I worked my way up to one-minute planks, three sets of ten lungs, thirty seconds jumping rope, and increasing my resistance bands to level two or three depending on the exercise, and intense floor exercises on the mat.

One exercise that is great for the lower abdominal is reverse crunches. Lie on your back on the mat and place your hands to your side, palm facing down and bring your knees towards your chest. Make sure you keep your feet together, hands stay palm-down, and you come up in a 90-degree angle. Hold your abs in tight to get the full effect of the crunch.

In the beginning, it was a nightmare. I had no idea how to perform a squat or lunge. Because of yoga, I knew how to do a chair pose. Like this:

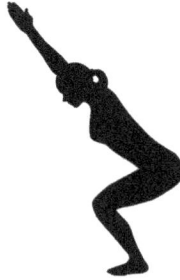

But squats, in which you crouch or sit with your knees bent and heels close to or touching your buttocks or the back of your thighs are different because you are going up and down.

For example, he would tell me to do three sets of ten squats and rest for two minutes between each set. I was like "what? Oh no. You're fired." Luckily, he had patience and enjoyed my humor, so this made it much easier.

We compromised, and I learned how to do squats using a chair, and I eventually graduated up to having the chair removed. I'm the squat queen now, but it took a month of me doing squats once a week to learn how to properly do a squat.

Great Benefits from a Personal Trainer

Hiring a trainer provided me the ability to learn about my body and what I was capable of achieving. My PT taught me that exercising is not about how fast you can go; it's about the technique. If you're lifting weights a hundred times the wrong way, and the person next to you is lifting weights fifty times the correct way, the person who lifts weights fifty times will see better results. This makes sense of course because the technique is correct and provides better results.

Health is Expensive

Switching over to a holistic lifestyle is not cheap. It all cost money. Aroma-therapy is expensive, as is getting a massage. And while doing yoga at home with a yoga tape is not costly, taking frequent classes at yoga studios is expensive.

Though I did save some money by hiring a new trainer, nevertheless it takes money to pay someone to come to your house and work with you one-on-one.

But that was another very valuable lesson: to learn that it's okay to invest in my health. Where I grew up if you hired someone to help you with your health or life you were conceited.

For this reason, my husband and family thought I was wasting my money. I knew it wasn't a waste because I was feeling and looking different. I was learning to enjoy life and look past my struggle.

The reality is we spend money on nice shoes, clothes, cars, and homes, and we invest little to nothing on our health or life. But our health and life are the most important instruments we have to navigate our world. Why not spend a few more dollars on your hair, nails, and exercise? Why not spend the time and exert the discipline needed to have peace of mind?

I was introduced to a group called *Dream Catchers* on Facebook, and this group taught me all about managing and investing in my finances. If you are searching for a book to help you with your budget, I suggest two:

The first is a very simple but straightforward way to get control of your spending: The Money Funnel System by Jaime and Cristina Farias. The other is *One Week Budget* by The Budgetnista, Tiffany Aliche. This is a great step-by-step guide on how to identify your budget and then manage it. I use this book as part of my health coach package because the majority of my clients suffer because of finances.

I now spare no expense when it comes to my health or peace of mind because it helps me be a better person. Our body is a temple of God, and we have to nurture and protect it to do God's work. This is my belief. Regardless if you have another belief, we can all agree you have to protect your body to be successful in achieving your goals.

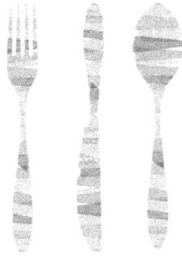

CHAPTER TWELVE

Getting a Divorce

No MATTER HOW MUCH WORK I DID ON MYSELF, HOWEVER, I KNEW THERE was something else that was not working in my life that needed attention.

After my mother's death and my son's heart transplant, it was clear I had to change the path I was on. I had done a good job really paying attention to the food I put in my body and the energy that created. Exercise was giving me a clear head to start the day with. But what about my relationships and the energy those were creating? In particular, I had to start with a relationship that was pulling me down and literally making me sick.

I met my husband when I was thirteen-years old. Yes, thirteen! We met through my niece's father. We talked for a few months, a lot on the phone—we were teenagers after all.

After a few years, he disappeared. He stopped calling and coming to visit, and I eventually moved on with my life. Right before I graduated from high school, he reappeared and we picked up where we left off. Talking every day. Going out to dinner on the weekends.

He was the perfect gentlemen and always treated me with respect. We used to laugh and have a good time together. My family liked him around and my mother, especially, thought the world of him. I was a teenager, into hanging out and partying, and she knew he could help me grow up and start to think about having a family.

Eventually we started a serious relationship; well, I thought it was serious. We moved in together and had our first baby when I was twenty-two. We were excited because our first born was a son.

I loved being a mom but felt the role alone was unfulfilling for me. I love to learn and grow and evolve. So I decided I needed to continue my education. I went back to school and received my degree. We finally got married when I was twenty-eight and he was thirty-years old.

Though my husband had a lot of good qualities and a lot of good existed in our relationship, there were major problems.

I believe he honestly didn't want to emotionally hurt me. Sometimes people do things out of low self-esteem that ends up hurting those they love without realizing the effect their behavior has on others.

Whatever my husband's motivations, I made the choice to marry him, and I now had to look myself in the mirror and ask why. When I did, I started to uncover a lot about who I was and to rethink everything in my life.

It wasn't about putting myself down and making myself feel bad but about facing the truth. And the truth was that I had been married for fourteen years and had been happy maybe four of the fourteen. That was it!

I was faced with making the decision to stay the same and possibly have an affair, which would have just been another unhappy relationship (and a sin at that, which would have gone against my principles) or to accept that I had made a bad decision and move on.

Obviously to have a better chance at happiness, I chose the latter. I was in an unhealthy marriage. If I loved and respected myself, it was time to move on. But I didn't end the marriage at that point.

Instead, I started doing things that made me happy. Most importantly, I worked on my spiritual self, making a point to go to church, pray, and meditate. These were the things that helped me centralize my emotions and focus on being the best me in life.

The more time I spent on making myself healthier and wiser, the less time I spent on worrying about what my husband was doing. I didn't do any of this to deliberately build my self-esteem, but that's what was happening. I was learning to love myself more and more.

None of this was easy. But I looked to God and he helped me understand what I needed to do within myself to be happy. And it wasn't yet time to leave my husband.

Instead of constantly disagreeing with my husband and fighting with myself about everything he wasn't going to be in my life, I decided to be a more loving, caring, and nurturing wife. Even though it wasn't mutual, I didn't care because it made me feel good and complete. It actually helped me learn more about myself.

I kept doing what I felt needed to be done for myself and my family. But I wasn't getting the message from God that it was time to divorce him. These thoughts were too scary. Instead, God was giving me the message to keep working on improving myself and in turn learning how to deal with the cares of life. That was enough for me at that moment.

Yoga helped as well. Yoga taught me to allow what felt natural to manifest in my life and not fight it. It is a woman's nature to be nurturing and caring. And that was my goal—at least for the time being.

And then one day, it all came crashing down. When I arrived home, my husband was gone. He had failed to take care of his responsibilities to the household. He told my son to tell me he was sorry and that he was leaving me.

Needless to say, that's when the marriage was over. God had moved him out of my life and I had to find the strength to move on without him.

When my husband walked away from the marriage, I knew that was the release I needed to be free and happy in my relationship goals.

Finally, I had a fresh start to create the healthy relationship I needed for balance and peace.

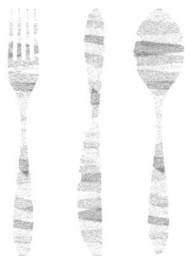

CHAPTER THIRTEEN

A Door Opens to A New Life

*"Let food be thy medicine
and medicine be thy food."*

~ HIPPOCRATES

I AM DETERMINED TO CONTINUE TO BUILD MY BODY, FUEL MY MIND, AND nourish my soul every day. When I made that decision, however, I also knew that I wasn't going to rush it. I realized that my goal was a lifetime quest, and I would take my time.

Life is a process. You have to understand yourself before you can truly understand what you want out of life. It takes time and involves digging through the hurt and joy in your life to understand the power of *me*.

Each day is a struggle as life without my thyroid gland will always present special challenges. I have good days, and I have bad days. I take in what is good and live out what is bad. Each day I meditate and focus on what works for me. I pay attention to what doesn't work for me, but I don't obsess on it. This helps me categorize my life and move towards a better me.

When I notice my hormone levels are off, I rest my body. I shut myself out from the world and pray, sleep, read, and eat fruits and vegetables until I start to feel my levels coming back to normal. Food *is* medicine and my diet allows this body to live! That's why I take care of it.

Finding this balance was not easy, and my life's journey has taken me off course many days and continues to take me off course. Some weeks, I'm down for a day or two, other times for a whole week. But I know how to fix it.

Intuitively, I know that when I ignore things in my life, my body shuts down and I feel horrible, and so I now know to acknowledge those feelings and situations that I used to pretend didn't exist. I will give it a moment or day to have its way while praying through the pain or joy. Eventually, my body will balance back out, and I start to feel better. Boy! I wish I had learned this in my twenties and thirties!

When I wake up, I say, "God you got me up this morning, so I'm expecting you to do great things in my life because you don't wake up failures."

I believe God wakes everyone up to be winners and allows us to decide if we are going to win or lose. Each day, I decide to win.

I'm not at the finish line, but I am no longer at the starting line. I have learned how to focus on myself—not in a selfish way, but in a focused way. I identify things that make me happy and appreciate the small things in my life. For example, I appreciated the ability to walk my dogs and enjoy the fresh air, the opportunity to sit on the park bench in the morning and read my daily word and pray. All this makes me so much more relaxed in life.

My children make me happy, and I enjoy seeing them smile. I raised some pretty awesome kids. They love me unconditionally, and they want to be great humans in this world.

My son is doing great with his new heart. He graduated from college and got a great job with the Department of Agriculture. My youngest son we call "smiley face boy" because he is always smiling. From the time he was a baby, he was smiling. I always say, "They belong to God and I'm just here to make sure they honor God and life."

Exercise makes me happy, and I enjoy how I feel and look. Of course, shopping makes me happy! And of course, cooking makes me happy, especially cooking my healthy vegetarian dishes.

After being alone for a while after my divorce, I started seeing a nice man. We married this past year, and you know what? I am happy with him! We have a loving, caring relationship based on mutual respect and trust. He is a blessing in so many ways.

And so I feel that I have achieved the biggest part of any of our lives—being happy and enjoying the life God gave us to live. It is a blessing just to know that my heart is working to bring me life and my lungs inhale and expire hundreds of times each day. I also know that at any time these organs can decide they've had enough of this work and will stop. Knowing this, I have learned to give thanks to each day. It is a joy to wake up and appreciate the gifts that God places in our path along the way. I'm learning each day to adjust to God's unchanging hand and this changing life we are living in.

My goal in writing this book was to heal my heart. In the journey of its production, I have learned to live a much healthier lifestyle. When you know better, you do better.

I know I don't have all the answers, and I could still become ill again. But I am going to do my best to feed my body foods that will help it thrive in this life. I am going to push my heart to live by exercising. I am going to harvest healthy relationships by pursuing happiness every day. I am going to stay in tune with my spirituality and the gift of life each day is a blessing not to be taken for granted!

It is almost cliché at this point to say that your body, mind, and spirit need to be aligned. Cliché's are dead, lifeless things. Living, however, has shown me that true balance between body, mind, and spirit is something that is in constant motion. Life is a constant striving to be better and do better in order to have a more fulfilling life.

There is no one "big goal" that I'm striving for either. Instead, it's the ability to live with joy each day and handle the barriers and struggles life throws in my way with grace and beauty. My health will never be perfect. I'm missing a vital piece that I'm constantly making up for. That doesn't stop me from living. If my story has inspired you to find a way to live not *in spite of* but *because of* the obstacles you face, then my work will not have been in vain.

I wish you well on your journey to a healthy body, mind, and spirit. Choose the path that is right for you in all respects. I chose God's path. You might find something different. But know that when you pay as much attention to your spiritual self as your physical self, things just seem to work better—sometimes a little, sometimes a lot. And isn't that all we can ask of ourselves and others, in the end?

About the Author

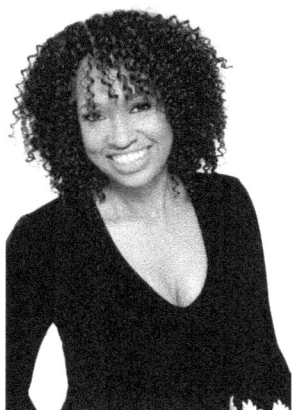

DESIREE GREEN DIDN'T START OUT AS A health coach. For the past two decades, she has been a program analyst, working her way into a supervisory role, but her life turned upside down when she was told she had to have her thyroid removed.

She took steroids, anti-depressants, and enough antibiotics to kill any germ. Nothing worked. Fed up watching the life she knew slip away, Green decided to take her health into her own hands. What she discovered changed her life. The healing Green experienced based on her own extensive research was so transformative that she felt she had been given a gift she must share with others.

Green is now a health coach specializing in holistic and herbal medicine and coaches others on the steps necessary to achieve lasting health and wellness in mind, soul, and body.

In *It Is Not About the Diet*, Green takes readers along with her on a journey of healing. She shares her initial struggles dealing with the mental and physical toll taken by thyroid disease, a condition that affects more than 20 million Americans. And she reveals a secret she learned along the way: that constant dieting will not help anyone with the mental and emotional issues that come from over and undereating. That there's a bigger picture of holistic healing that can only start when root causes are addressed.

For the millions of people around the world suffering from today's modern plagues—mental illness, obesity, metabolic disease, autoimmunity, thyroid disease, and more—there is hope! Green's mission is to help others discover what it takes to find balance and live an active and healthy life, using the techniques she has discovered that help her manage her own health and stay well, including yoga, essential oils, herbal remedies and much more.

Follow Desiree Green on social media at:

- Instagram: @naturaltrinityblog
- Twitter: @natltriblog
- Facebook: @naturaltrinity
- Web: naturaltrinity.com

www.ingramcontent.com/pod-product-compliance
Lightning Source LLC
Chambersburg PA
CBHW022340280326
41934CB00006B/720